PRAISE FOR
HIPAA DEMYSTIFIED

"HIPAA compliance is so much more than just passing out the Notice of Privacy Practices at the first client contact. In *HIPAA Demystified*, Dr. Lorna Hecker explains the essence of the Health Insurance Portability Accountability Act of 1996 and translates it in an understandable manner, allowing readers smooth implementation of the regulations to their practices. Each chapter is arranged with clarifying 'demystification' summaries that explain HIPAA requirements in actionable terms. Dr. Hecker's use of real world case examples illustrating breaches of protected patient health information reminds us how easily this can happen and how to mitigate those risks. Search no longer, *HIPAA Demystified* will be your ultimate guide to HIPAA compliance."

Norman C. Dasenbrook, MS, LCPC
Practice Consultant
Dasenbrook Consulting
Rockford, IL.

"HIPAA is becoming the standard of care for mental health, whether or not one is officially a 'covered entity'. Therefore, it is critical that all mental health practitioners, and mental health programs and agencies, understand and adhere to the standards of care under HIPAA. While maintaining confidentiality is integral to training and practice, protecting the security of information is less familiar, and there is a need for resources that address this gap in literature. *HIPAA Demystified: HIPAA Compliance for Mental Health Professionals* meets this need and is a practical and readable resource. Clearly explaining the regulations and law, Dr. Hecker leads the reader to answer pertinent questions to develop a step-by-step guide to implementing a customized compliance program. Key to providing safeguards is a risk assessment, and the book guides you in doing so. Dr. Hecker discusses many critical elements for a mental health practice, such as clarification of how a psychotherapy note is defined by HIPAA and what other types of information are not considered psychotherapy notes. Real world examples throughout the book illustrate the complex set of Privacy and Security Rules applicable to mental health, thus helping the reader establish safeguards to avoid breaches. A model Notice of Privacy Practices is provided as well as numerous links to websites relevant to navigating the HIPAA road! Overall, this book is an extremely relevant and helpful resource for mental health professionals who strive to maintain the security of protected health information while navigating rapidly changing technologies."

Mary K. Alvord, Ph.D.
Psychologist and Director, Alvord, Baker & Associates, LLC
Adjunct Associate Professor of Psychiatry and Behavioral Sciences
at The George Washington University School of Medicine and Health
Sciences, Rockville, MD

"*HIPAA Demystified* provides a superb opportunity for professionals in an agency or corporate setting to more comprehensively assess risk. Through the understanding of changing technologies, Dr. Hecker affords readers the opportunity to more globally understand the aspects of their agency that must be scrutinized. In an agency setting, the opportunity to identify and mitigate areas of concern is truly paramount. The agencies involved in mental/behavioral health treatment often have to find creative ways to survive, thrive, and maintain revenue streams in today's insurance driven marketplace. Any seminal event can lead to devastating legal and financial consequences. Not only does this book help to identify the legal ramifications that could impact an organization of any size, but it also sheds light on the financial outcomes that could be debilitating. A thorough assessment and understanding of the necessary HIPPAA guidelines allows for an agency to avoid financial hardship brought about by the results of damaged reputation, diminished patient care, and weakened organizational and funding source partnerships.

HIPAA Demystified brings to light the necessity of thoroughly understanding the reach of risk assumed within an agency. Without this book, risk through areas such as subcontractors or other extensions of business will be difficult to pinpoint. Dr. Hecker thoughtfully allows for readers to gain a comprehensive understanding of the differing types of risk and the impact associated with it. Agencies are only as strong as their weakest link, and therefore the need for training is of the utmost importance. *HIPAA Demystified* informs the necessity of training at every level of the organization. Overall, *HIPAA Demystified*, was insightful, informative, well written, and thought-provoking. A must read for any professional, from student to CEO."

Daniel Lettenberger-Klein M.S., LMFT
Regional Service Director
Sunrise Detox
Alpharetta GA

"Hecker has created a fantastic resource for new graduates and seasoned mental health practitioners alike. This practical guide to HIPAA compliance efficiently breaks down the components of healthcare privacy into palatable pieces, informing readers without overwhelming. Hecker provides contemporary examples throughout the book to illustrate the true impact of privacy breaches, bringing the importance of thorough compliance to life. *HIPAA Demystified* is the resource to keep on hand as you navigate the complexities of patient privacy in this digital era"

Christine Borst, PhD, LMFT
Director of Operations
Center of Excellence for Integrated Care
Cary, NC

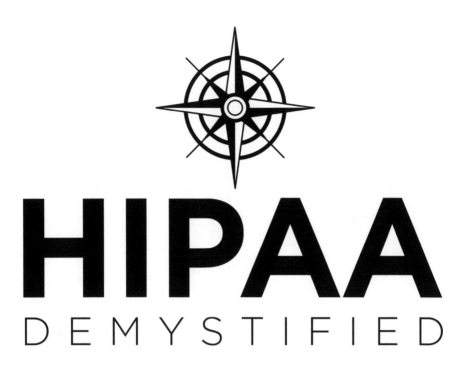

HIPAA

DEMYSTIFIED

HIPAA Compliance for
Mental Health Professionals

LORNA HECKER, PH.D.

TABLE OF CONTENTS

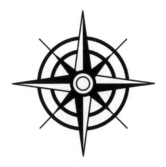

PREFACE

Confidentiality is the ethical obligation of a mental health practitioner to keep patient information private; we respect this obligation due to our moral and professional values, ethical codes, and state statutes. Privacy is the right of clients to be free from the intrusion of others into their personal life. Both confidentiality and privacy are important foundations to psychotherapy practice. However, as we move into an era of electronic health records (EHRs), we must delve into a new area of confidentiality and privacy, which is the security of electronic records and other forms of digital data we maintain on our patients. With the advent of EHRs, the federal government realized that the public would have concerns about the privacy of this electronically kept personal health information. The Health Insurance Portability and Accountability Act (HIPAA) of 1996 was enacted, bringing federal uniformity to protecting the privacy of paper health records, as well as protecting the security of electronic health information. HIPAA gave patients[1] additional rights about the uses and disclosures of their private health information, as outlined in the familiar Notice of Privacy Practices, typically given on a patient's first visit. But what is HIPAA beyond this notice? Many practitioners are still confused about HIPAA requirements. This is understandable given there are over 1,500 pages of HIPAA regulations, detailing privacy requirements, security requirements, and electronic data interchange requirements. The advent of the Health Information Technology

1

for Economic and Clinical Health (HITECH) Act, enacted in 2003, brought even more requirements including breach notification regulations.

There are some regulations of which most mental health practitioners have limited knowledge. Here are a few for you to check your knowledge base:

- Do you understand the HIPAA definition of psychotherapy notes?

- Have you completed a security risk assessment and produced a remediation plan based on the results?

- Do you understand what is required of you if a patient asks for an accounting of disclosures?

- Do you understand the difference between a designated record set and a legal record set?

- Have you designated a privacy official and a security official in your practice?

- Have you integrated stricter state standards[2] into your Notice of Privacy Practices?

- Do you understand the process of breach, a risk analysis in the event of a breach, and breach notification requirements?

- Have you instituted a workforce sanction policy, detailing potential consequences for HIPAA violations?

- Do you have a way to stay abreast of recent HIPAA developments, such as the 2013 revision requirements for your Notice of Privacy Practices?

If you can answer these questions affirmatively, congratulations, you are ahead of the curve! If you thought having a Notice of Privacy Practices and HIPAA-compliant software made you compliant, you have a ways to go. This book will help you take stock of your HIPAA compliance, demystifying the requirements such that you can more readily adapt them in your practice. Additionally, you will find case scenarios on breach of protected health information based on actual cases such that you can learn from the mistakes of others. After reading this book and implementing the regulations that apply to your practice, you will be much more confident in pronouncing to your patients that you are indeed in compliance with the regulations.

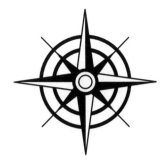

CHAPTER 1
Introduction to HIPAA Compliance

While mental health professionals are intimately familiar with patient confidentiality,[3] security of patient information in the digital arena has been limited or ignored. Yet, patients are rightfully concerned about the security of their health information remaining private and secure. Identity theft of personal information may result in criminals opening new telephone service accounts, credit cards, loans, checking and savings accounts, and online payment accounts. Medical identity theft is increasing with stolen identities used to procure medical treatment, services, and supplies. Additional dangers may lurk when a patient's records later reflect incorrect medications or medical conditions.[4] Thieves have been known to give stolen identity information to law enforcement when they are stopped or charged with a crime; rent housing; obtain government benefits; or obtain employment, medical or mental health treatment, services, or supplies.[5] Tax fraud is also of concern. The digital tsunami of the past few decades has not been met with equal force in protection of our most personal data. Mental health professionals who value confidentiality must also learn to value security of the electronic health data they collect on patients in order to keep patient trust.

History and Purposes of HIPAA

Congress passed the Health Insurance Portability and Accountability Act (HIPAA) in 1996 with two general purposes. The first was to ensure that individuals could maintain health insurance between jobs (portability), and the second was designed to ensure privacy and confidentiality of patient health information (accountability). Under Title II of HIPAA, Administrative Simplification, the government addressed this accountability by developing privacy and security regulations. The Privacy Rule requires appropriate safeguards to protect privacy of health information and sets limits and conditions on the uses and disclosures that may be made of an individual's health information.[6] The Privacy Rule was created to lessen inappropriate disclosure of Protected Health Information (PHI) and give individuals increased control over their PHI. The Security Rule protects an individual's Electronic Protected Health Information (EPHI), providing safeguards to protect the confidentiality, integrity, and security of that digital data[7] that is created, received, used, or maintained by a provider.

Title II of HIPAA, Administrative Simplification, is directly applicable to psychotherapy practice. It includes the Privacy and Security Rules, as well as standards around electronic data interchange. In 2009, the American Reinvestment and Recovery Act (ARRA) brought the Health Information Technology for Economic and Clinical Health (HITECH) Act, which strengthened HIPAA. HITECH established breach notification rules, increased restrictions on disclosures of PHI, gave patients more rights regarding their PHI, increased fines and established criminal penalties for violations of HIPAA regulations, and provided certain other restrictions. HITECH also brought resources for compliance audits, which as a result are occurring more frequently.

Protected Health Information (PHI) is any health information that can be used to identify a patient, who relates to physical or mental health, relating to a past, present, or future condition, and includes both living and deceased patients.[8] PHI may be in any form: Oral, paper, or electronic (transmitted and maintained).

Compliance with HIPAA Regulations

HIPAA compliance means that you have followed the HIPAA and the HITECH Act federal regulations set by the Department of Health and Human Services (HHS) and enforced by the Office of Civil Rights (OCR). Many companies promise HIPAA compliance, yet there is no such thing; HHS does not grant compliance to entities or companies. Software vendors and others cannot apply for approval and become "HIPAA compliant." The reality is you must manage your ongoing compliance with the entirety of the privacy and security regulations consistently over time. This requires knowledge of the regulations, acquiring and applying updates when the regulations change, keeping up on evolving technology and weaknesses of your current technology infrastructure, ongoing training for your workforce, and so on. The goal of HIPAA compliance is to protect the privacy and security of your patient's private, confidential information, including any spoken, written, and electronic information.

HIPAA DEMYSTIFIED

Companies that promise you HIPAA compliance are not being entirely candid. The truth is, compliance efforts to protect the privacy and security of patient protected health information are ongoing. For example, your vendor cannot rely on an accrediting agency to certify that they are HIPAA compliant or certify that no one would be able to hack their system. It is your responsibility to assess their level of compliance under the HIPAA regulations and the level of risk you are taking on through the use of their service. Only you can create privacy and security for your clients through ongoing efforts to safeguard protected health information.

Noncompliance with HIPAA Regulations

Violations of HIPAA regulations are, unfortunately, commonplace. The extent of HIPAA violations ranges from unintentional disclosure to willful disclosure for personal gain (i.e., criminal enterprise). HIPAA violations largely went unpunished until the HITECH Act of 2009 clarified fines and penalties for HIPAA violations. The OCR, the branch of the HHS that investigates HIPAA violations, began compliance audits and began instituting fines and penalties for violations. Noncompliance means not following the regulations, which can result in a breach of PHI. *Breach* refers to the acquisition, access, use, or disclosure of PHI that compromises the security or privacy of the PHI. Certain breaches of PHI result in the OCR levying fines; penalties may be brought through the Department of Justice. Breaches may even garner news coverage due to breach notification rules. For large breaches, patients must be notified, news media must also be notified, and details of the breach must be posted on the organization's website. Covered Entities (CEs) must self-report breaches to HHS; Business

Associates (BAs) must self-report breaches to the CE who contracted them. Failure to self-report can be seen as "willfull neglect," which results in additional fines. Because of these reporting measures, we are increasingly hearing about breaches of PHI. Public notifications, fines, penalties, and audits have all pushed breach of PHI to the top of the news.

The amount and depth of PHI breaches is staggering. In 2015, hackers stole PHI of 8.8 to 18.8 million people by hacking the database of Anthem Blue Cross Blue Shield.[9] Shortly after the Anthem breach, Premera Blue Cross was hacked, breaching the personal and health data of 11 million members.[10] While mental health information was surely included in these breaches, stand-alone mental health organizations have also seen significant breaches and fines. A few examples include the following:

- The nonprofit community mental health center Aspire Indiana lost the health data of 45,000 patients after several laptops were stolen from their offices.[11]

- A company laptop and hard drive of Arizona Counseling and Treatment Services were stolen from an employee's home, resulting in the loss of health data of more than 500 patients.[12]

- Compass Health, a behavioral health organization in Washington, lost a laptop containing PHI including clinical data.[13]

- The HMO Harvard Community Health Plan had electronic notes of psychotherapy sessions available in its database to which all employees had access.[14]

- Comprehensive Psychological Services in South Carolina had a laptop stolen, which included psychological records and custody evaluations.[15]

Fines and Penalties for Noncompliance

There are four categories of HIPAA violations that reflect increasing levels of culpability, paired with four corresponding tiers of penalty amounts. Fines range from $100 to $50,000 per violation with a $1.5 million cap for all violations of an identical provision in a calendar year. If violations resulted from "willful neglect," which is conscious, unintentional failure, or indifference to the obligation, there are mandatory fines of $10,000 to $50,000. Offenses committed with the intent to sell, transfer, or use PHI for commercial advantage, personal gain, or malicious harm have the highest fines and terms of imprisonments. Criminal penalties may include fines and/or imprisonment from one to 10 years, dependent upon the level of mal-intent.

HIPAA DEMYSTIFIED

Costs of noncompliance with HIPAA regulations can include fines and penalties from the Department of Health and Human Services, but also include other types of financial losses, reputational damage, ethico-legal costs (e.g. harm to patients, legal liability), and damage to the therapist–patient relationship. You can spend far more in direct and indirect costs than you will on compliance efforts! Additionally, intentionally ignoring the regulations requires mandatory fines ranging from $10,000 to $50,000. Using protected health information for nefarious purposes can also garner jail time. Table 1.1 and Table 1.2 summarize civil and criminal penalties.

There are four categories of violations that reflect increasing levels of culpability and four corresponding tiers of penalty amounts that increase the minimum penalty amount of $1.5 million for all violations of identical provisions. Penalties are lowest if a CE did not know and with reasonable diligence would not have known about the violation. Additionally, penalties are waived for any violation that is corrected within a 30-day time period, as long as the violation was not due to willful neglect (e.g., ignoring the regulations).

HIPAA Violation	Minimum Penalty	Maximum Penalty
Individual did not know and by exercising due diligence would not have known (and was generally diligent in following HIPAA regulations)	$100 to $50,000 per violation. No penalty if corrected within 30 days. Fees may be waived or penalties reduced by OCR.	Annual maximum of $1.5 million for identical provisions in calendar year
HIPAA violation due to reasonable cause (not due to willful neglect)	$1,000 to $50,000 per violation. No penalty if corrected within 30 days. OCR can waive or reduce penalties.	Annual maximum of $1.5 million for identical provisions in calendar year
HIPAA violation due to willful neglect (but violation remediated within the required time period)	$10,000 to $50,000 per violation. Penalties mandatory. This category of willful neglect occurs only when the violation is corrected within 30 days after the covered entity knew, or should have known that the violation occurred.	Annual maximum of $1.5 million for identical provisions in calendar year
HIPAA violation due to willful neglect (and is not remediated)	$50,000 minimum per violation minimum per violation.	Annual maximum of $1.5 million for identical provisions in calendar year

Table 1.1. Civil fines for HIPAA violations (these figures represent fine schedules after February 18, 2009)

HIPAA Violation	Financial Penalty	Criminal Penalty
Knowingly and wrongfully used and/or disclosed PHI	Fine up to $50,000	Imprisonment up to one year
Deceptively used and/or disclosed PHI (false pretenses)	Fine up to $100,000	Imprisonment up to five years
Used PHI for profit or false pretenses (with intent to use for personal gain or malicious harm or to sell, transfer, or use for commercial advantage)	Fine up to $250,000	Imprisonment up to 10 years

Table 1.2. Criminal fines and penalties for HIPAA violations (these figures represent fine schedules after February 18, 2009)

Fines. Violations of HIPAA regulations may lead to fines ranging from $100 per violation/record to $50,000 per violation, with an annual maximum of $1 million. For example:

- Anchorage Community Mental Health Services was required to pay $150,000 to the HHS after it failed to patch its data systems, ran outdated software, and had a breach of 2,743 records. HHS stated that it had failed to identify and address basic security risks.[16]

- Affinity Health Plan Inc. was fined $1,215,780 when it returned multiple photocopiers to a leasing agent without erasing the data contained on the copier hard drives.[17]

- The Alaska Department of Health and Human Services was fined $1,700,000 when it failed to take corrective action to improve its policies and procedures after a USB drive was stolen from the vehicle of an employee.[18]

Penalties. There is an increasing roster of individuals who are being charged with criminal penalties including fines and jail time. In these cases, the offender has mal-intent. For example:

- When a doctor in Los Angeles was fired, he decided to read confidential medical records of both his supervisor and high-profile celebrities. He was sentenced to four months in prison and fined $2,000.[19]

- A nurse in Arkansas accessed a patient's file and shared the information with her husband who planned to use it in a legal proceeding. She was sentenced to two years' probation and 100 hours of community service.[20]

- A former hospital employee in Texas was sentenced to federal prison for 18 months for selling patient PHI for personal gain.[21]

Additional Costs of HIPAA Violations

For the average practitioner, there are additional costs for HIPAA violations. These include additional financial costs, reputational costs, legal, ethico-legal costs, and potential loss of patients due to damage to the therapeutic relationship.

Financial. The evolving standard practice in response to breaches is that the violating entity pays for ID theft / credit monitoring for patients whose PHI was breached. Financial loss may include image repair for public relations efforts, workforce sanctions (e.g., firing), or change in vendors when a BA is responsible for the breach. Loss may also include loss of current patients, loss of future patients, loss of customers (those who pay for services), loss of new business, and loss of staff. The American National Standards Institute (ANSI) estimates the percentage of lost revenue by the magnitude of breach. It estimates an insignificant breach costs less than 2% of revenue, a minor breach is 2% of revenue, a moderate breach is 4% of revenue, a major breach is 6% of revenue, and a severe breach will cost more than 6% of revenue.[22] The Ponemon Institute notes that costs for a data breach to be around $200 per individual record.[23]

Reputational. Breaches that affect over 500 individuals are to be reported to HHS and must be reported "without reasonable delay", and at the latest 60 days from first learning about the breach. Your name or your practice's name, type of breach, and number of people affected gets posted to the HHS website, to an area colloquially known as the "Wall of Shame." Additionally, patients and local media are to be notified, and breach information is to be posted on the practices' website.

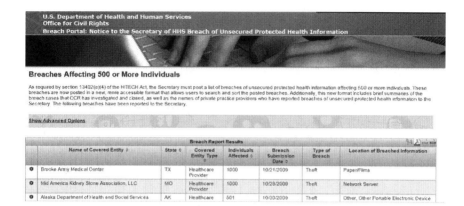

The HIPAA "Wall of Shame" Breach Portal[24]

Ethico-Legal. The requirements of the privacy and security regulations have become the standard of care for both physical and mental health professionals.[25] If your HIPAA compliance is below par, harm to patients and legal liabilities can occur. For example, when medical identity fraud has occurred, fraudulent claims may be processed, diagnoses may be delayed or inaccurate, and insurance benefits exhausted.

While there is no private cause of action written in HIPAA regulations, (e.g., you can't be sued for violating HIPAA) other types of legal action can occur in the event of a breach of PHI. You may be subject to state breach notification requirements, state consumer protection laws, or civil lawsuits for privacy violations. Under HIPAA regulations, a state's attorney general may take legal action for HIPAA violations. Accreditation bodies may also sanction your practice for violations of the regulations. Lastly, HIPAA is beginning to be used in lawsuits as the standard of care for privacy and security of PHI (*c.f. Acosta v. Byrum* [26]).

Patient–Therapist Relationship. Concerns about privacy also affect the therapeutic relationship. In one study, 45% of patients surveyed said they were "very" or "moderately" concerned about their medical records or insurance information being accessed without their consent. The same survey noted that a whopping 21% of patients withheld theirs or their family's mental illness, substance abuse history, and prescription information from the treatment provider due to privacy concerns.

———•———————————————•———

"But I have a small practice—is HIPAA really important?" In 2011, Hospice of North Idaho was required to pay $50,000 for a breach of 441 records due to a stolen laptop. Upon investigation, the Office for Civil Rights found that it had not done a required security risk assessment and it had no HIPAA policies and procedures in place for mobile device security.[27]

Indeed, most breaches occur within small practices. Patient confidentiality no longer lies solely by guarding what you say and to whom you say it, or safeguarding paper files. The digital era has ushered in a new type of vigilance required to protect private client information, with specific parameters provided by HIPAA regulations.

———•———————————————•———

Determining if HIPAA Applies to Your Practice

If you practice, furnish, bill, or receive payment for healthcare in your normal course of business, or if you provide services to someone who does, you are likely bound to comply with HIPAA regulations. Individuals, organizations, or agencies that meet the definition of a CE need to comply with the privacy and security regulations. BAs are entities that perform functions or activities on behalf of CEs, involving use or disclosure of PHI. BAs and subcontractors of BAs need to comply with the security regulations, and any contracted privacy requirements.

Covered Entities

A CE is any entity that transmits any information in an electronic form in connection with a transaction for which HHS has adopted a standard. Most commonly for practitioners, the main trigger for HIPAA compliance is filing for insurance reimbursement, or reimbursement from government funding entities such as medicare or medicaid. Individuals or organizations are considered CEs only if they transmit information in an electronic form in connection with a transaction as designated by HIPAA.

There are three categories of CEs: healthcare providers, health plans, and healthcare clearinghouses.

Healthcare Providers. Healthcare providers include doctors, clinics, mental health professionals, dentists, chiropractors, nursing homes, and pharmacies, physical therapists, rehabilitation practitioners, dieticians, occupational therapists, medical laboratory clinicians, among others.

Health Plans. Health plans include health insurance companies, HMOs, company health plans, or government programs that pay for healthcare such as Medicare, Medicaid, or military or veteran's healthcare programs.

Healthcare Clearinghouses. Healthcare clearinghouses (HCCs) are entities that receive healthcare transactions from healthcare providers or other third-party payers and then translate the data into a format that is accepted for payer(s). HCCs may also be an entity that receives this data and then processes the information into a nonstandard format, relating to claims and billing information.

Hybrid Entities. In addition, there is a lesser-known CE, a hybrid entity. A hybrid entity is an organization that has both covered and non-covered functions. For example, at a university a counseling center or healthcare center may meet the requirements to be a CE, but other parts of the university do not (e.g., physics, history). Those parts of the hybrid entity that provide covered functions must comply with HIPAA regulations.

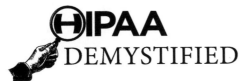

HIPAA
DEMYSTIFIED

If you do electronic billing *for even one patient*, you are considered a covered entity. If you subsequently opt out of electronic billing that previously triggered HIPAA, you must keep documentation of your previous HIPAA compliance for six years after the last electronic transaction.

Business Associates and Subcontractors

A BA is an entity or organization that creates, receives, maintains, transmits or stores PHI on behalf of a CE. Examples include entities who process claims, provide billing services, perform data analysis, or practice management. BAs may also be entities that provide legal, actuarial, accounting, consulting, data aggregation, management, administrative, accreditation, or financial services for a CE if the service involves the disclosure of PHI. For mental health practitioners, this typically includes your billing service, answering service, attorneys, outside consultants who have access to PHI, shredding and documentation companies, and so on. A CE may also find that it is also a BA in the event that it creates, receives, maintains, transmits, or stores PHI for another CE.

BAs are required to maintain the privacy and security of PHI as provided by their business associate agreements (BAAs) or other written contracts.

With the advent of the HITECH Act of 2009, BAs are required to comply with breach notification requirements and are subject to the same civil and criminal penalties as CEs. A BA may have some interaction with your patients; they must disclose PHI when a patient or the representative requests the PHI through the CE. Due diligence must be performed to gain satisfactory assurances that a CE's BAs are complying with HIPAA regulations. BAs must assure that any of their subcontractors are also complying with the regulations.

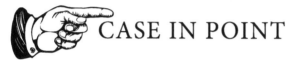 CASE IN POINT

Clyde's Counseling, a HIPAA covered entity, uses Betty's Billing service. Because Betty's Billing service handles receipts and billing statements, creates authorization reports, follows and verifies insurance benefits including PHI, Betty's Billing is considered a business associate under the regulations. Betty's Billing gathers a lot of protected health information paperwork in the course of business and must confidentially dispose of some protected health information from time to time. Betty's Billing hires Sam's Shredding service. Because Sam's Shredding is also handling the protected health information of Clyde's Counseling, Sam's Shredding is considered a subcontractor of Betty's Billing.

If a BA subcontracts part of its function whereby another entity creates, receives, maintains, transmits or stores PHI on behalf of a CE, the subcontractor is also subject to HIPAA security regulations, as well as any privacy stipulations set by the BA. BAs and their subcontractors are not required to name privacy officials for their organization, but must designate a security official. While BAs and their subcontractors do not have to comply with the privacy regulations, they are bound by their

Business Associate Agreements (BAAs). In these agreements, CEs will likely stipulate compliance with many of the privacy regulations. For example, if a BA keeps treatment records, and a patient wishes to amend those records, the BA must comply with this aspect of the privacy regulations. When CE requirements are discussed in this book, they typically also apply to BAs, with few exceptions.

HIPAA DEMYSTIFIED

Nearly every practitioner is a covered entity, business associate, or subcontractor of a business associate, and subject to HIPAA regulations. For those few practitioners or practices that do not meet the criteria that trigger the need to be compliant with HIPAA regulations, state statutes may still cause practitioners to be subject to similar privacy and security regulations. If your practice does not meet the criteria to be a covered entity, know that many states now have breach notification laws and typically have stronger privacy statutes around mental health treatment that require vigilance to oral, written, and electronic protected health information. Case law is also beginning to establish HIPAA regulations as the standard of care for privacy and security of protected health information.

Compliance Audits

Lastly, the HITECH Act requires the Office for Civil Rights (OCR) to perform audits, which are increasing in frequency, even for smaller providers. Both CEs and BAs can be subject to an audit. A breach is not a prerequisite for an audit. During the first phase of audits in 2011–2012, 58 of the 59 CEs had a security finding (i.e., noncompliance). Most commonly,

CEs were simply unaware of HIPAA requirements. Two-thirds of CEs had not done the required security risk assessment; small providers (10 to 50 provider practices) struggled the most with compliance.[29] HHS is using the monies they take in from fines and penalties, in part, to further their audit efforts. Therefore, auditing will continue to increase; mental health practitioners are not immune. The audit process begins with an email from OCR asking for documentation regarding your compliance (e.g. HIPAA policies and procedures). You have 10 days to respond to the email and submit your documentation to the OCR. Your business associates may also be audited. An on-site visit by OCR may be required.

Summary

HIPAA was created in 1996; Title II, Administrative Simplification, affects most practitioners. Title II brought forth privacy and security regulations. CEs are required to follow the privacy and security regulations. BAs are required to follow the security regulations, and any privacy regulation stipulations set by the CE. HHS is responsible for overseeing implementation of HIPAA regulations, while the OCR is responsible for enforcing the privacy and security regulations. Noncompliance with HIPAA regulations can bring fines and penalties, with further consequences such as financial, reputational, ethico-legal problems, and damage to the therapist–patient relationship. HITECH funding for compliance audits is increasing the amount and frequency of audits, including for mental health practitioners. The purpose of this book is to guide mental health practitioners who are CEs and BAs (or their subcontractors) through HIPAA regulations to increase HIPAA compliance, thereby increasing patient confidence in the privacy and security of their personal information in which they entrust you, their provider.

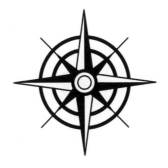

CHAPTER 2
HIPAA and Mental Health

Mental health professionals covered under HIPAA regulations must abide by all of the regulations that any other healthcare provider does. However, psychotherapy notes receive special attention within the regulations. Recognizing the need for higher protection of mental health information, the Department of Health and Human Services (HHS) specifically defines and protects a practitioner's psychotherapy notes. This is both good and bad news. Fortunately, patients have been granted federal protection for their psychotherapy notes from compelled disclosure, reinforcing federal protection of privilege set by *Jaffee vs Redmond* [30] Unfortunately, what is included in the definition of psychotherapy notes is fairly limited.

Psychotherapy Notes (45 CFR §164.508)

Psychotherapy notes are uniquely defined by HIPAA regulations and differ from more general information in a patient's file. Psychotherapy notes are often referred to as *process notes* or sometimes *personal notes*. They are to be kept separate from the medical (i.e., case) record and are given special protection because they contain sensitive information that is relevant to no one other than the practitioner.

The HIPAA definition of *psychotherapy notes* is "notes recorded (in any medium) by a health care provider who is a mental health professional documenting or analyzing the contents of conversation during a private counseling session or a group, joint, or family counseling session and that are separated from the rest of the individual's medical record."[31]

Psychotherapy notes:

- include the practitioner's impression of the patient

- include details of the psychotherapy session inappropriate for the medical record

- are solely for the use of the practitioner, for example, for planning future sessions

- are kept separate to limit access (including in an electronic health record [EHR]).

To qualify for special protections under HIPAA, psychotherapy notes are to be maintained separately from the medical record and must be maintained solely by the originator of the notes. They cannot be used to substantiate billing, and need not be in a particular format (such as handwritten). If psychotherapy notes are kept, another note documenting the service must be kept for billing and legal purposes. Psychotherapy notes may be accessed only by the practitioner or, depending upon the practice, possibly a supervisor. No other staff can access these notes. For electronic health records, this is typically accomplished by having a section of the chart that is hidden and accessed only with an individual password. Psychotherapy notes are not offered heightened protection in the following situations:

- If psychotherapy notes are kept in a second location, they are not eligible for heightened protection under the regulations. For example, in a group practice, if a practitioner keeps a second set of psychotherapy notes others may access, the second set of psychotherapy notes does not have heightened protection.

- If a patient requests that psychotherapy notes be released to another party or to themselves, once the notes are released they are no longer afforded special protection under HIPAA regulations.

- Testing may reveal sensitive information but does not qualify for heightened protections.

- If your practice is part of an integrated health network and psychotherapy notes are routinely shared with others in the network, they are not psychotherapy notes as defined by HIPAA regulations.

Under HIPAA regulations, psychotherapy notes do not have to be shared with clients unless required by state law. A denial of access to psychotherapy notes is not appealable under HIPAA regulations.

(H)IPAA DEMYSTIFIED

Psychotherapy notes are finally afforded federal protection; however psychotherapy notes are narrowly defined and do not include all patient protected health information. State laws may also be relevant in defining psychotherapy notes. HIPAA regulations do not require practitioners to keep psychotherapy notes. Additionally, practitioners are not compelled to share psychotherapy notes with patients under HIPAA regulations, unless state law stipulates their release.

Information Not Considered Psychotherapy Notes (45 CFR §164.501)

What other types of information are *not* considered psychotherapy notes? The following information is not considered to be psychotherapy notes and does not receive a higher level of protection than other types of health information (PHI):

- summary information, such as the current state of the patient
- summary of the theme of the psychotherapy session
- medications prescribed and side effects (if applicable)
- any other information necessary for treatment or payment (e.g., PHI routinely sent to insurers for payment)
- current state of the patient
- treatment plan, symptoms, and progress
- diagnoses and prognosis
- counseling session start and stop times
- the modalities and frequencies of treatment furnished
- results of clinical tests
- any other information necessary for treatment or payment.

A patient's insurance company may have access to this information, but it is not privy to psychotherapy notes. PHI, besides the specifically defined psychotherapy notes, may be disclosed without a separate authorization form signed by the patient or the representative. The patient is asked to sign an acknowledgement of a Notice of Privacy Practices (NPP) when services commence but is not required to give specific authorization for release of anything other than the psychotherapy notes when it is used for treatment, payment, or healthcare operations (physical health may require an authorization to release certain other medical information). State law typically provides heightened restrictions regarding release of mental health information, as do professional codes of ethics.

Use and Disclosure of PHI in Mental Health Practice (45 CFR §164.506)

Under HIPAA, there is a regulatory difference between use and disclosure of PHI. *Use* includes the sharing, application, use, examination, or analysis of PHI within your organization. *Disclosure* refers to the release of, transfer of, provision of, access to, or divulging of PHI in any other manner to any outside entity. The privacy regulations detail both uses and disclosures of PHI.

Practitioners may use and disclose PHI to other providers involved in the patient's care about medical file information without an authorization when it is for treatment, payment, or healthcare operations (TPO), but not about the specific content of the psychotherapy notes unless there is patient authorization. This means that as a CE, summary information including the current state of the patient, treatment plan, symptoms, progress, diagnoses, etc. can be shared with others involved in TPO. *Treatment* includes consultation between providers. *Payment* refers to payment or reimbursement (e.g., claim submission, authorizations, and payment postings), and healthcare *Operations* include quality assessment, competency assessment, performance evaluations, credentialing audits, and so on.

Generally, any disclosure of information that is not for TPO requires an authorization. When sharing information pursuant to an authorization, the information you share must be the minimum necessary to accomplish the intended purpose (there are some situations where the minimum necessary standard does not apply, such as when information is needed for treatment purposes. This will be addressed in detail in chapter 4).

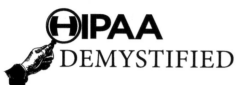

Any protected health information that is for treatment, payment, or health care operations (TPO) may be released without an authorization. Under HIPAA regulations psychotherapy information may be released without an authorization, psychotherapy notes may not. This can get confusing; remember there is a difference between what goes into the chart as more general psychotherapy information (e.g., dates of treatment, treatment plan, session start and stop times), versus what is kept privately by the therapist as psychotherapy notes. State laws regarding sharing of mental health information may be stricter, which protects mental health information from release without written authorization. Many states, however, allow sharing of mental health information for TPO. States also typically allow sharing of protected health information in the case of emergency. To add to the confusion, mental health professional codes of ethics often prohibit sharing of protected health information. Practitioners should access an attorney familiar with mental health law to work out the specifics to their practice's confidentiality policies and procedures.

When Psychotherapy Notes May Be Disclosed Without an Authorization (45 CFR §164.512)

There are a few exceptions whereby psychotherapy notes can be disclosed without authorization under the regulations. These include:

- for your own training or supervision
- for defense in legal proceedings brought by the individual

- for HHS to investigate or determine the CE's compliance with the Privacy Rules

- to avert a serious and imminent threat to public health or safety (e.g., abuse reporting, duty to warn, duty to protect)

- to a health oversight agency for lawful oversight of the originator of the psychotherapy notes

- for the lawful activities of a coroner or medical examiner or as required by law.

Practitioners must manage different types of disclosures of PHI: some governed by HIPAA, some by state law, and some by professional codes of ethics. Practitioners typically obtain a release of information to disclose PHI to others outside of therapy; state law often governs this. Under HIPAA regulations, a release of information is not needed to divulge psychotherapy information for purposes of TPO. This is considered "use" of PHI; patients are informed of this potential use in the NPP (to be described in chapter 4) with the exception of psychotherapy notes, for which you need a HIPAA-compliant authorization. You are required to give patients a NPP and attempt to obtain their signature acknowledging receipt of the notice. This acknowledgement signature can be part of your overall patient consent to treatment or can be obtained on a separate acknowledgement form. If a patient refuses to sign the acknowledgement, you are required to document the refusal, but you may not withhold services soley due to the refusal to sign the acknowledgement. Due to this stipulation, the acknowledgment may best be separated from the informed consent.

Understanding Notices, Authorizations, Informed Consent, and Disclosure Statements

To clarify, various ways practitioners may release information: A HIPAA CE is required to give the patient an NPP, notifying patients of their rights and how a CE will use or disclosure their PHI. If releasing psychotherapy notes, there must be a patient authorization (state law may also dictate the content of a patient authorization in addition to HIPAA requirements). Typically, practitioners ask clients to sign an informed consent to inform the client of the risk and benefits of treatment, office policies, and so on. Most states require a disclosure statement, which is minimally a statement of the psychotherapist's educational and training background, but each state has its own specific requirements for these documents. See Table 2.1 for a summary of various types of notices and consents typically needed for mental health treatment.

Type of Disclosure	Definition	Who Requires?	Signature Needed?
Notice of Privacy Practices	Describes permitted uses and disclosures of PHI	HIPAA	A good faith effort to obtain signature must be made
Patient Authorization	Permission to use PHI for specific non-TPO purposes (e.g., psychotherapy notes)	HIPAA	Yes
Informed Consent	Describes risks and benefits of treatment (as well as other relevant treatment information)	Professional codes of ethics; some states may have additional requirements	Yes
Disclosure Statement	A document given to patients that minimally describes a psychotherapist's training and education; further requirements set by state law	State governed; requirements vary by state	Typically not, but is often included as part of informed consent

Table 2.1. Types of notices and consents that may be needed for mental health treatment

While an authorization for release of information is not needed for TPO, an authorization is needed to release information if it is *not* for TPO. Psychotherapy notes always require an authorization. HIPAA allows requests for disclosure of PHI to be made by mail, email, or fax or in person. The exception to release of PHI occurs when a patient pays out of pocket. In this case, the patient has the right to request that the provider not report or disclose individually identifiable information or PHI to health insurers, with some limitations (to be described in chapter 4).

Components of a HIPAA-Compliant Authorization (45 CFR §164.508)

HIPAA requires specific elements to be included in an authorization. Authorizations need to include:

- a specific description of health information to be disclosed
- name of person or organization authorized to release the information
- name of person authorized to receive the information
- a description of each purpose of the requested disclosure
- an expiration date or event
- signature of the patient or legal representative
- a statement that the patient has a right to revoke the authorization in writing
- a statement that the patient's treatment or payment could not be conditioned on their permission to release private information
- a statement of the potential for re-disclosure of the information by the recipient
- the form must be written in plain language.

Authorizations are prohibited if submitted documentation has an expiration date that has passed, if the form has not been filled out completely, if a CE knew the authorization has been revoked, or if the CE knows the information on the form is false.

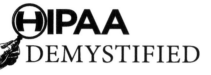

Under HIPAA regulations there is specific verbiage that must be included in your authorizations. In addition to HIPAA regulations, you may have state regulations regarding how an authorization must be written. If there is discrepancy between state law and HIPAA regulations, the more strict law applies (i.e., the law that gives patients more control over their protected health information).

Ability to Establish Stricter Policies

HIPAA regulations establish a floor for privacy protections. It does not prevent you from establishing a policy that the patient (or their representative) provides consent on disclosures that would otherwise be allowed by HIPAA. There should be an inclusion of any provisions of state law or in the NPP.

HIPAA and State Law (45 C.F.R.§160.202)

States commonly have special confidentiality protection for mental health records that are more stringent than HIPAA. *More stringent* means either that the law provides more privacy protections for a patient or that the patient has greater access or rights regarding health information. Additionally, if a professional code of ethics overrides HIPAA, necessitating consent before records are released, you may follow your code of ethics. However, some professional codes of ethics have language that client confidences are to be up held except where mandated or permitted by law. State law may narrow the scope or duration of the authorization, in which case state law should be followed information on a particular state law can be found at http://www.alllaw.com/state_resources.

Let's imagine a state law allows patients to access their psychotherapy notes; HIPAA does not. State law is to be followed as HIPAA states the law with greater patient rights prevails. In this case, if a patient requests psychotherapy notes in a state that allows access, then that request is to be honored.

For example, in Minnesota, individuals have the right to view or release all parts of their medical records (psychotherapy notes are considered part of the medical record in Minnesota, even if kept separately from the medical record).[32] Thus, in Minnesota, state law gives the patient more rights and supersedes HIPAA.

In Virginia, there is no designation for psychotherapy notes; all mental health information is treated as medical information. Thus, in Virginia, state law also gives the patient rights to their medical information and a patient would be able to see their psychotherapy notes.

What is confounding is that state laws do not always define *psychotherapy notes* or they have other names for psychotherapy notes (e.g., personal notes). Not all states differentiate between mental health records and medical records. However, states are attempting to clarify right of access. For example, Wisconsin has clarified that *treatment records* do not include notes or records for personal use by the practitioner; thus, they are not part of the legal health record or designated record set (to be defined and discussed in chapter 6) and are therefore are inaccessible to patients.

Clarification of HIPAA regulations in comparison to state law will continue to evolve as states make policy statements or where case law has established precedent. For now, it remains rather murky because state mental health laws vary in their definitions of mental health / psychotherapy notes. Most states, however, do allow the practitioner to withhold notes if they believe their release to the patient would be harmful in some way.[33]

Keep in mind that access to records is not the only issue that must be analyzed between the state and federal levels. State release of records (authorization) criteria need to be compared to HIPAA authorization criteria, searching for the more stringent option. HIPAA always preempts state law in these areas:

- preventing fraud and abuse
- state reporting of healthcare delivery or costs
- ensuring appropriate state regulation of insurance and health plans
- addressing controlled substances
- reporting of disease or injury
- child abuse, birth, or death
- public health surveillance, investigation, or intervention
- other purposes as outlined by HIPAA law.

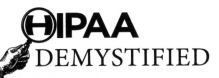

HIPAA
DEMYSTIFIED

When weighing HIPAA and state regulations, the law that gives patients greater privacy protections or greater access rights is the law to be followed. However, there is nothing to prevent a practitioner from establishing practice policies that give further privacy protections to clients, though protected health information must be disclosed when legally required.

Additional Federal Regulations

In addition to HIPAA regulations, practitioners may fall into more than one "camp" of regulations, with differing requirements. For example, those who are HIPAA compliant, depending upon practice, may also have to be compliant with the Medicaid or Medicare regulations, the Family Educational Rights and Privacy Act (FERPA), the Federal Confidentiality of Alcohol and Drug Abuse Patient Records regulations (42 CFR Pt 2), the Gramm-Leach Bliley Act (personal financial information), Sarbanes-Oxley (financial reporting), or the payment card industry data security standard (credit card security). If part of a Health Information Exchange, the larger organization may have regulations if it received "meaningful use" monies that were distributed under the American Recovery and Reinvestment Act (ARRA) to facilitate the adoption of electronic medical records. These regulations may alter the stipulations for consents and authorizations. If bound under several regulations, you typically follow the more strict law. Ambiguities occur as illustrated in the "Case in Point" that follows.

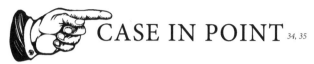

CASE IN POINT [34, 35]

At times, laws are ambiguous, leaving practitioners with little guidance. For example, HIPAA regulations explicitly state that protected health information excludes any individually identifiable health information in educational records covered by the Family Education Rights and Privacy Act (FERPA). Controversy erupted in 2015 when a student at the University of Oregon alleged three university basketball players raped her. She sued the university for mishandling her rape. She had previously been seen in counseling at the university health center. In preparing for the lawsuit, the university accessed the student's mental health records from her counseling sessions at the university. Uproar ensued; while the health center is a HIPAA covered entity, because the regulations specifically exclude FERPA covered information, the stronger privacy protections did not prevail. Concerned that college students have less privacy rights than the general public, an Oregon senator and representative have asked the Department of Education clarify its records policy as a result.

Electronic Data Interchange / Covered Transactions
(45 CFR §160 and 45 CFR §162)

Mental health practitioners typically encounter HIPAA electronic data interchange (EDI) regulations when they bill third-party payers for services rendered. The HIPAA EDI regulations established national health transaction standards and code sets for covered transactions. A covered transaction under HIPAA is an electronic transmission of healthcare claims, payment, remittance, benefit, or health plan eligibility information. EDI originated as a way to standardize the claims processing and payment cycle and the eligibility and payment cycle. This information is often handled between Healthcare Clearinghouses (HCCs) and third-party payers.

Healthcare Clearinghouses (45 CFR §164.104)

To get reimbursed for services, practitioners must submit claims to payers (e.g., insurance), with an appropriate procedure and diagnosis code(s). HCCs are entities that take a provider's claims for reimbursement and "scrub" them. Scrubbing is cleaning of the claim to be sure that it is appropriate for submission and subsequently reimbursement. This may mean correcting data-entry errors and making sure that the codes and modifiers meet payer guidelines or verifying that the codes and diagnoses are compatible. Software used to submit the claim is compatible with the payer's software. HIPAA regulations require that the transmission between payers and providers be standardized; thus, an HCC acts as the intermediary between payers and providers and transfers information using standard formats set by the regulations.

In the unlikely event that you are an HCC and part of a larger organization, you must implement policies and procedures to protect the electronic PHI from unauthorized access by others within the organization, as any CE would protect PHI from outside entities.

Coding for Claims (45 CFR §162.1000)

Mental health professionals typically submit claims using ICD (International Classification of Diseases), and CPT (Current Procedural Terminology) codes. While HIPAA requires standard transactions and code sets with the goal of increasing speed and accuracy of claims processing, most practitioners will tell you that reimbursement is a moving target and is far from a smooth process.

Unique Identifiers (45 CFR Part §162.406)

EDI includes the use of unique user identifications for providers, employers, and health plans. The goal of unique identifiers is to facilitate processing of claims and enrollment. There are three types of unique identifiers:

1. **National Provider Identifier.** The national provider identifier (NPI) is used in administrative and financial transactions. A 10-digit numeric identifier assigned to each healthcare provider. Provider IDs can be obtained through the National Plan and Provider Enumerator System. Provider IDs may be assigned to individuals or organizations.

2. **Standard Unique Employer IDs.** A 9-digit employer identification numbers (EIN) is assigned by the IRS. The EIN must be used in standard transactions between payers and providers, this is also referred to as the federal tax identification number.

3. **Health Plan Identifier.** A 9-digit unique Health Plan Identifier (HPID) is assigned to each health plan.

While the government originally intended for there to be a unique patient identification number, ironically, it has not come to fruition because of privacy concerns.

Summary

HIPAA has given a federal boost to the privacy of psychotherapy notes, buttressing the *Jaffee v. Redmond* U.S. Supreme Court decision[36] that established privilege for therapy communications in the federal courts; without a doubt at the federal level, there is an understanding that psychotherapy communications need to be kept confidential. Conversely, HIPAA narrowly defined what is to be given a higher level of protection are "psychotherapy notes," which have a limited definition and leave much client information available to both the courts and other inquiries (e.g., diagnoses, treatment plan, symptoms, test results). Further, patient information, with the exception of psychotherapy notes, can be freely transmitted for TPO, unless state law prohibits it. The untangling of state law from HIPAA regulations can be challenging. Unless there are federal preemptions, state laws that give patients more privacy protections or access rights should be followed.

In an effort to standardize payment transactions, promote efficiency, and encourage the use of electronic health records, HIPAA adapted EDI standards, affecting healthcare claims, payment, remittance, benefit, or health plan eligibility information. For mental health professionals, healthcare claims are often handled by a billing service, which deals with the HCCs. Unique identifiers such as an NPI and standard unique employer identification (EIN) are used for processing purposes.

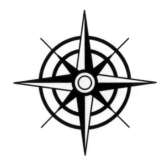

CHAPTER 3
Introduction to the Privacy Regulations

Privacy within HIPAA focuses on an individual's right to maintain one's health information in a protected way. The Department of Health and Human Services (HHS) was charged with establishing regulations to protect patient privacy. The Office of Civil Rights (OCR) is responsible for implementing and enforcing the Privacy Rule. The Health Information Technology for Economic and Clinical Health (HITECH) Act further buttressed the privacy regulations with increased enforcement efforts and a breach notification rule.

The Privacy Rule established national standards to protect patient records and other patient information for providers who conduct certain transactions electronically. Privacy within HIPAA relates to both living and deceased patients and can be related to a past, present, or future condition. The Privacy Rule gives patient's rights around their Protected Health Information (PHI).

Privacy Rule Standards[37]

Throughout the next two chapters, the standards of the Privacy Rule will be discussed. All standards in the Privacy Rule are required; they *must* be implemented. A summary of the Privacy Rule standards follows:

Requirement	Standards
45 CFR §164.502 Uses and Disclosures of PHI	45 CFR §164.502(a) A covered entity may not use or disclose PHI, except as permitted or required by the regulations
	45 CFR §164.502(b) Minimum necessary
	45 CFR §164.502(c) Uses and disclosures of PHI subject to an agreed-upon restriction
	45 CFR §164.502(d) Uses and disclosures of de-identified PHI
	45 CFR §164.502(e) Disclosure to business associates
	45 CFR §164.502(f) Deceased individuals
	45 CFR §164.502(g) Personal representatives
	45 CFR §164.502(h) Confidential communications
	45 CFR §164.502(i) Uses and disclosures consistent with notice
	45 CFR §164.502(j) Disclosures by whistleblowers and workforce member crime victims
45 CFR §164.504 Uses and disclosures: Organizational requirements	45 CFR §164.504(e)(1) Business associate contracts
	45 CFR §164.504(f)(1) Requirements for group health plans
	45 CFR §164.504(g) Requirements for a covered entity with multiple covered functions
45 CFR §164.506 Uses and disclosures to carry out treatment, payment, or healthcare operations	45 CFR §164.506(a) Permitted uses and disclosures

Requirement	Standards
	45 CFR §164.506(b) Consent for uses and disclosures permitted
45 CFR §164.508 Uses and disclosures for which authorization is required	45 CFR §164.508(a) Authorizations for uses and disclosures
45 CFR §164.510 Uses and disclosures requiring an opportunity for the individual to agree or object	45 CFR §164.510(a) Uses and disclosure for facility directories
	45 CFR §164.510(b) Uses and disclosures for involvement in the individual's care and notification
45 CFR §164.512 Uses and disclosures for which an authorization or opportunity to agree or object is not required	45 CFR §164.512(a) Uses and disclosures for which an authorization or opportunity to agree or object is not required
	45 CFR §164.512(b) Uses and disclosures for public health activities
	45 CFR §164.512(c) Disclosures about victims of abuse, neglect, or domestic violence
	45 CFR §164.512(d) Uses and disclosures for health oversight activities
	45 CFR §164.512(e) Disclosures for judicial and administrative proceedings
	45 CFR §164.512(f) Disclosures for law enforcement purposes
	45 CFR §164.512(g) Uses and disclosures about decedents
	45 CFR §164.512(h) Uses and disclosures for cadaveric organ, eye, or tissue donation purposes
	45 CFR §164.512(i) Uses and disclosures for research purposes

Requirement	Standards
	45 CFR §164.512(j) Uses and disclosures to avert a serious threat to health or safety
	45 CFR §164.512(k) Uses and disclosures for specialized government functions
	45 CFR §164512(l) Disclosures for workers' compensation
45 CFR §164.514 Other requirements relating to uses and disclosures of PHI	45 CFR §164.514(a), (b), and (c) De-identification of PHI
	45 CFR §164.514(d) Minimum necessary requirements
	45 CFR §164.514(e) Limited data set
	45 CFR §164.514(f) Uses and disclosures for fundraising
	45 CFR §164.514(g) Uses and disclosures for underwriting and related purposes
	45 CFR §164.514(h) Verification requirements
45 CFR §164.520 Notice of Privacy Practices for PHI	45 CFR §164.520(a) Notice of Privacy Practices for PHI
45 CFR §164.522 Rights to request privacy protection for PHI	45 CFR §164.522(a) Right on an individual to request restriction and disclosures of their PHI
	45 CFR §164.522(b) Confidential communications requirements
45 CFR §164.526 Amendment of PHI	45 CFR §164.526(a) Right to amend
45 CFR §164.528 Accounting of disclosures of PHI	45 CFR §164.528(a) Right to an accounting of disclosures
45 CFR §164.530 Administrative requirements	45 CFR §164.530(a) Personnel designations
	45 CFR §164.530(b) Training

Requirement	Standards
	45 CFR §164.530(c) Safeguards
	45 CFR §164.530(d) Complaints to the covered entity
	45 CFR §164.530(e) Sanctions
	45 CFR §164.530(f) Mitigation
	45 CFR §164.530(g) Refraining from intimidating or retaliatory acts
	45 CFR §164.530(h) Waiver of rights
	45 CFR §164.530(i) Policies and procedures
	45 CFR §164.530(j) Documentation
	45 CFR §164.530(k) Group health plans

Table 3.1. Privacy Rule standards

Summary

The HIPAA Privacy Rule brought federal protections to individually identifiable health information held by CEs and their BAs. The Privacy Rule was designed to be balanced between the need to have access to health information and the need for individual privacy. Definition and exploration of each of the Privacy Rules required for HIPAA compliance follow in the next three chapters. CEs must comply with the Privacy Rule; BAs must comply with the privacy regulations as stipulated in the business associate agreement.

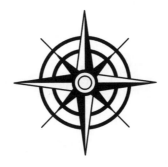

CHAPTER 4

Uses and Disclosures of
Protected Health Information

Within HIPAA regulations, "use" of Protected Health Information (PHI) refers to the sharing, employment, application, use, examination, or analysis of such information within an entity that maintains such information. "Disclosure" of PHI means the sharing, employment, application, utilization, examination, or analysis of such information within an entity that maintains such information (45 CFR §160.103). Under HIPAA regulations, PHI may be used (within a practice) and disclosed (outside of a practice) for treatment, payment, and healthcare operations (TPO) (45 CFR §164.506(a)). One of the goals of HIPAA is to make coordination of services easier; thus the regulations allow sharing of treatment information for TPO purposes. HIPAA specifies when disclosures are restricted or permitted and enforces a "minimum necessary standard" to limit what is used or disclosed to the minimum information necessary to accomplish the intended purpose.

Patients have a right to know how and to whom their PHI is being shared, which is detailed for them in the Notice of Privacy Practices (NPP). Consent (acknowledgement of practices designated in the NPP) is not sufficient for disclosing PHI when it is not for TPO; an authorization is necessary (45 CFR §164.506(b)). The regulations also specify what disclosures require an authorization, and who may authorize these disclosures. Authorizations are not needed when PHI is de-identified or limited data sets are used, as is the case for research or operations purposes (to be discussed below). Authorization is always needed for the release of psychotherapy notes. A covered entity (CE) may not use or disclose PHI except as permitted or required by the regulations (CFR 45 §164.502). In this chapter, we discuss permitted uses and disclosures of PHI as well as specific prohibitions against disclosures under the Privacy Rule.

Minimum Necessary Standard (45 CFR §164.502(b); 45 CFR §164.514(d))

A CE must make reasonable efforts to limit information release of PHI. The minimum necessary standard (MNS) indicates PHI should not be used or disclosed when it is not necessary to satisfy a particular purpose or carry out a function. For routine or recurring disclosures, it is advised that policies and procedures be established that outline the minimum necessary requirements for those disclosures.

Some CEs facilitate the MNS by using one of three types of access to EPHI. They are:

- user-based access: a person is allowed access based on who they are
- role-based access: a person is allowed access based on what their job function is
- context-based access: a person is allowed access based on where the user accesses data.

The MNS does not apply when the PHI is needed for treatment, when the patient requests information or they (or their personal representative) have authorized release, or when the Department of Health and Human Services (HHS) needs access for complaints or compliance audits. When another CE requests PHI, you are allowed to rely on the request of other

CEs or Business Associates (BAs), public officials, professionals such as attorneys or accountants, and researchers to be the minimum necessary needed for their purposes. When evaluating the MNS, it is helpful to think of these questions: Is the information needed for my job? How much information do I need to know? How much do other people need to know to do their job? CEs must develop policies and procedures around identifying the persons or classes of persons who need access to PHI to carry out their duties. It is best to establish standard protocols for routine, recurring disclosures.

(H)IPAA
DEMYSTIFIED

When responding to a request for information, you must limit disclosures to the *minimum necessary* to accomplish the intended purpose. The minimum necessary standard does not apply with protected health information is needed for treatment purposes, or when patients or their personal representative have authorized release, or if required by the Department of Health and Human Services.

Permitted Disclosures

HIPAA allows the release of PHI in certain cases without having to obtain a patient's consent. In some situations, absolutely no authorization is required. In others, while no written consent is required, a practitioner must give the patient the opportunity to agree or object to the disclosure.

Disclosures When No Authorization Is Required

(45 CFR §164.501; 45 CFR §164.502)

CEs may use or disclose PHI without obtaining an individuals' authorization or offering the ability to agree or object to the disclosure in the following circumstances.

- to the individual who is the subject of the information (45 CFR §164.524) (except psychotherapy notes)

- for TPO (45 CFR §164.506)

- for incidental use and disclosure (this includes many customary healthcare communications such as calling a patient's name in the waiting room) (45 CFR §164.502(a)(1)(iii))

- for public interest and benefit activities, which include:

  o those required by law (45 CFR §164.512(a))

  o public health activities (45 CFR §164.512(b)) (e.g., communicable disease)

  o authorities regarding victims of abuse, neglect, or domestic violence (45 CFR §164.512(c)). Note: a CE who makes this disclosure must promptly inform the individual that such a report has been made unless the CE believes that it would put the individual at risk of harm, if a CE believes that the personal representative is responsible for the abuse, neglect, or other injury

  o health oversight activities (45 CFR §164.512(d)) (e.g., government benefits oversight)

  o judicial and administrative proceedings (e.g., court order) (45 CFR §164.512(e)) PHI may be disclosed in response to an order of a court or other adjudicative entities, provided that the CE discloses only the PHI expressly authorized by such order. Satisfactory assurance should be obtained that the individual has been informed of the disclosure, and had the opportunity to object. Alternately, the CE may inform the individual of the request prior to disclosure.

- o lawful enforcement purposes (45 CFR §164.512(f)). This may include limited information for identification purposes, about a victim of a crime, someone who has died, or a crime on premises or reporting of a crime
- o regarding decedents (e.g., to funeral directors) (45 CFR §164.512(g))
- o cadaveric organ, eye, or tissue donation (45 CFR §164.512(h))
- o research purposes (45 CFR §164.512(i)) (when approved by IRB or a privacy board)
- o serious threat to the health or safety to a person or to the public (45 CFR §164.512(j)) (e.g., prevent harm)
- o essential government functions (e.g., national security purposes) (45 CFR §164.512(k))
- o worker's compensation (45 CFR §164.512(l))

- when disclosing de-identified data (to be discussed later in this chapter). If the health information meets the de-identified standards, it is not considered individually identifiable heath information (e.g., not PHI) and may be used and disclosed (45 CFR §164.514(a))

- when using a limited data set (LDS) if the disclosure is for research purposes. An LDS is PHI from which specified direct identifiers of individuals and their significant others and place of employment have been removed: dates, ZIP code, and the city or town remain (45 CFR §164.514(e))

- for fundraising, certain PHI may be released to a BA or institutionally related foundation. PHI that may be released for fundraising includes demographic information relating to the patient including name, address, other contact information, age, gender, and date of birth. Additional inclusions that are allowed are dates of service, department where the patient was seen, treating physician, outcome information, and health insurance status. However, the patient must be notified of fundraising activities in the Notice of Privacy Practices. Each fundraising activity must include an opt-out from further fundraising communications, as well as a method to opt back in (45 CFR §164.514(f))

- for underwriting purposes. If certain criteria is met, a health plan may use PHI for underwriting, premiums ratings, or other activities related to health insurance plans (45 CFR §164.514(g))

- disclosures to BAs (45 CFR §164.502(e)). A BA is a person or organization that performs work for a CE that involves access to PHI. A BA can also be a subcontractor responsible for creating, receiving, maintaining, transmitting, or storing PHI on behalf of another BA. If a CE enlists the help of a BA, a written contract or other arrangement between the two must be in place (the BA contract will be discussed in detail in Chapter 12). Common BAs for practitioners are the billing company, consultants, and attorneys. A CE can also be the BA of another CE. Prior to this disclosure, a CE must obtain satisfactory assurances that the BA will appropriately safeguard all of this information. CEs are not required to obtain assurances for any subcontractors of the BA; the BA must obtain the assurances from the subcontractor.

Disclosures Requiring an Opportunity to Agree or Object (45 CFR §164.510)

Practitioners may disclose PHI provided that the individual is informed in advance and given the opportunity to agree or object to the disclosure (or limit the disclosure). In other words, if a client gives oral agreement to any of the following, a written authorization is not needed:

- An individual's name, location, general condition, religious affiliation may be listed in a directory (e.g., hospital directory) if the individual does not object.

- Under emergency circumstances, PHI may be given unless the provider knows the individual's wishes have previously been expressed and are to the contrary, and the provider determines it is in the individual's best interests.

- PHI may be revealed to those involved with an individual's care, such as a family member, other relative, or close personal friend of the individual, or any other person identified by the individuals, the PHI directly relevant to the person's involvement with the individual's healthcare or payment.

- If an individual is present, PHI may be disclosed if the individual agrees, if the individual has had have had the opportunity to object, or the provider reasonably infers from the circumstances that the individual does not object to the disclosure.

- A CE may use or disclose PHI to notify or assist in notification (including identifying or locating) a family member, a personal representative, or person responsible for the care of the individual, the individual's location, general condition, or death.

- If an individual is not present, and the opportunity to agree or object cannot be obtained due to incapacitation or emergency circumstance, the CE may disclose PHI directly relevant to the person's care, payment of the care, or for notification purposes.

- A CE may also use or disclose PHI in the event of a disaster, to a public or private entity to assist in disaster relief efforts.

- If an individual is deceased, a CE may notify a family member, personal representative, or other person involved with the individual's healthcare or payment for that healthcare of the death of the individual, unless this has been previously prohibited by the individual.

Again, while HIPAA regulations allow for communication of this information, the state law may be more stringent and therefore apply unless there is a federal pre-emption. This state law may reside in mental health statutes or can also be found in medical records statutes.

Prohibited Uses and Disclosures (45 CFR §164.502 (a)(5))

PHI may not be sold or marketed without a specific authorization, and PHI may not be used or disclosed for genetic information underwriting purposes.

Verification Requirements (45 CFR §164.514(h))

Before disclosing PHI, a CE must verify the identity of the person requesting the PHI, and the authority the person has to access the PHI. The CE needs to obtain satisfactory assurances that the person to whom they are releasing the PHI is authorized to receive it. This includes release to public officials such as law enforcement, who can verify with their identification badge or other official credentials or proof of government status. CEs are expected to exercise professional judgement when making decisions about release of PHI.

Requests for Restrictions of Uses and Disclosures
(45 CFR §164.502; 45 CFR §164.522(a))

Individuals have the right to request a CE restrict use or disclosure of PHI for TPO. Patients may also request to restrict disclosure to persons involved in their care or payment for their care or disclosure to notify family members or others about the individual's general condition, location, or death. Requests must be submitted in writing. A CE does not need to agree to these requests for restrictions. If a CE does agree to restrictions, it must comply except for purposes of treatment during a medical emergency. In an organized healthcare arrangement (OHCA), participating CEs may share PHI to manage and benefit the OHCA. A restriction must be documented, with a copy of the documentation retained for six years from the date the restriction was created or last effective (whichever is later).

Restrictions will not be honored when information is needed for the following reasons:

- is investigating HIPAA compliance by the CE
- for public health activities
- concerning victims of abuse, neglect, or domestic violence
- health oversight activities
- for judicial or administrative proceedings
- to avert a serious threat to health or safety
- for worker's compensation and specialized government functions
- as required by law.

Requests for Confidential Communications (45 CFR §164.502(h))

Patients have the right to request an alternative means or location to receive confidential communications about their healthcare. For example, they may request appointment reminders be sent via email. Reasonable requests should be accommodated. Patients also have the right to request that you not release their information to their health insurer, *if* they pay out of pocket, request the restriction, and the restriction is not legally prohibited.

Disclosures Regarding Deceased Individuals (45 CFR §164.502(f))

While the length of the time required to keeping records is a state statute issue, if records are retained, privacy must be maintained as per the regulations for a period of 50 years following the death of an individual.

Disclosures to Personal Representatives (45 CFR §164.502(g))

A CE may give personal representatives the same rights they would the patient themselves. Regarding treatment and records of minors, in most cases parents (or persons acting in loco parentis) are the personal representative and can access medical information for their child. However, the Privacy Rule defers to state and other laws to determine parental access. Many states specify parental access to mental health information. If state law is silent, a CE has discretion to use its professional judgment to provide or deny a parent treatment information.

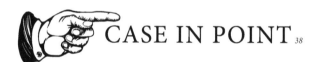 **CASE IN POINT** [38]

A mental health center did not provide an Notice of Privacy Practices to the father of a minor daughter. The Office for Civil Rights investigated, and the center acknowledged that it had not provided the father the notice prior to her mental health evaluation. The center revised its intake assessment policies and procedures to specify that the center provide the notice at intake and attempt to obtain a signed acknowledgement. The center also promised to train the staff on these privacy practices.

Whistleblowers and Victims of Crime
(45 CFR §164.502(h); 45 CFR §164.502(j))

A CE must comply with privacy regulations when communicating PHI (45 CFR §164.502(h)), consistent with the NPP, to be discussed in chapter 5 (45 CFR §164.502(i)). HIPAA allows for disclosure of PHI for whistleblowers, or if a workforce member is a victim of a crime (45 CFR §164.502(j)), they may divulge PHI to a law enforcement official if the PHI is about the suspected perpetrator of the crime, using the minimum necessary standard.

Optional Consent for Permitted Uses and Disclosures (45 CFR §164.506(b))

While not required, CEs may obtain consent from an individual (patient or their personal representative) to use or disclose PHI to carry out TPO.

Disclosures for Which an Authorization Is Required (45 CFR 164.508(a))

An authorization is always required for the release of psychotherapy notes, as well as for the marketing and sale of PHI.

Psychotherapy Notes (45 CFR §164.508(a)(2)). Disclosure of psychotherapy notes always requires a written authorization. Sharing of psychotherapy notes and other mental health treatment information may be restricted by state law. All state laws allow some flexibility during emergencies, and many allow sharing of PHI for TPO.

Marketing & Sale of PHI (45 CFR 164.508(a)(3); 45 CFR 164.508(a)(4)). PHI to be used for marketing and sale of PHI also requires an authorization (45 CFR §164.508(a)(3)). The marketing restriction does not include standard information about your practice, or small advertising trinkets you may wish to give to clients or the public.

De-identified Data and Limited Data Sets
(45 CFR §502(d); 45 CFR §164.514)

The Privacy Rule protects all "individually identifiable health information," which is either health information that identifies an individual, or there is a reasonable basis to believe the information can be used to identify the individual. There are three categories of individually identifiable health information (IIHI) that must be considered when contemplating using and disclosing IIHI: (1) PHI, which includes 18 individually identifiable health information identifiers (which will be described in detail below); (2) de-identified data, which has the 18 individually identifiable health information identifiers stripped from it so that it is no longer considered PHI; and (3) a limited data set, whereby 16 individually identifiable health identifiers need to be removed and a data-use agreement must be in place with any entity accessing the information. The purpose of de-identified data or a limited data set is that the information may be used for research, public health, or healthcare operations without specific patient authorization.

18 Identifiers of PHI (45 CFR)

PHI includes any information that can be used to identify an individual that relates to their past, present, or future health. There are 18 identifiers that make health data PHI; without them, health information by itself is not considered PHI. That is, if any of the following 18 identifiers are connected to health data, it is considered PHI and protected under the regulations:

1. Names
2. All geographic subdivisions smaller than a state including street address, city, county, precinct, ZIP code (and their equivalent geographical codes), except for the initial three digits of a ZIP code if, according to the current publicly available data from the Bureau of the Census:
   a. the geographic unit formed by combining all ZIP codes with the same three initial digits contains more than 20,000 people
   b. the initial three digits of a ZIP code for all such geographic units containing 20,000 or fewer people are changed to 000
3. All elements of dates (except year) for dates directly related to an individual including birth date, admission date, discharge date, date of death; and all ages over 89 and all elements of dates (including year) indicative of such age, except that such ages and elements may be aggregated into a single category of age 90 or older
4. Telephone numbers
5. Facsimile numbers
6. Electronic mail addresses
7. Social security numbers
8. Medical record numbers
9. Health plan beneficiary numbers
10. Account numbers
11. Certificate/license numbers
12. Vehicle identifiers and serial numbers including license plate numbers
13. Device identifiers and serial numbers
14. Web universal resource locators (URLs)
15. Internet protocol (IP) address numbers
16. Biometric identifiers including fingerprints and voiceprints
17. Full-face photographic images and any comparable images
18. Any other unique identifying number, characteristic, or code, unless otherwise permitted by the Privacy Rule for re-identification.

De-identified Data

There are three ways to de-identify data to where it is no longer considered PHI. The first is the Safe Harbor method, the second is the Expert Method, and the third is through a Limited Data Set. De-identified data may be used for research, marketing, and business development purposes, among others.

Safe Harbor Method. It is considered "safe harbor" when all 18 identifiers have been removed from health data. Once the 18 identifiers are stripped *and* there is no reasonable basis to believe that it could identify an individual, it is considered de-identified.

Expert Method. In this method, de-identify data is when an expert (e.g., a statistician), evaluates the risk of identification and, using statistical procedures, certifies that the risk of data being linked to a patient is negligible.

Limited Data Set. An LDS is still considered PHI but has certain identifiers removed and allows use of PHI for research, public health, or healthcare operations. All PHI must be stripped from the data except: dates such as admission, discharge, service, date of birth or death, city, state, five digit or more zip code; and ages in years, months or days or hours. A data use agreement must be in place with the entity using the PHI.

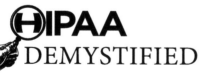

All protected health information requires a release if it does not fall under the classification of treatment, payment, or healthcare operations (with some legal exceptions). A limited data set may be released for research purposes with a data-use agreement. De-identified data may be used or disclosed without an authorization;

it is typically used for research, marketing, or other business or healthcare purposes. De-identified data has 18 protected health information identifiers removed such that the information may not be linked to a patient. A qualified statistician may also certify risk of data being linked to a patient is negligible in order for health information to be considered de-identified.

Administrative Requirements (45 CFR §164.530)

There are particular administrative requirements for the privacy regulations. These include the following:

- **Privacy Official** (45 CFR §164.530(a)(1)). A CE must designate a privacy official who oversees development and implementation of the Privacy Rules; a contact person or office must be designated.

- **Training** (45 CFR §164.530(b)). A CE must train all workforce members with respect to PHI such that they can carry out their duties and when there are material changes required, training must occur within a reasonable period of time. Training must be documented; new workforce must be trained within a reasonable period of time. Training occurs when policies or procedures change, when HIPAA regulations change, or when there is a breach of PHI. Otherwise, training occurs in regular intervals, typically yearly.

- **Safeguards** (45 CFR §164.530(c)). A CE must have in place appropriate administrative, physical, and technical safeguards to protect the privacy of PHI, and limit incidental uses disclosures pursuant to an otherwise permitted or required use or disclosure. It is a good idea to include your paper PHI in your electronic security risk assessment, to be covered in chapter 8.

- **Complaints** (45 CFR §164.530(d)). A CE must have a process in place for individuals to make complaints concerning the CE's policies and procedures protecting their PHI; the complaint documentation must be kept, as well as the CEs response to the complaint, if any (for six years).

- **Sanctions** (45 CFR §164.530(e)). A CE must apply appropriate sanctions when the workforce fails to comply with privacy policies and procedures of the CE. Applied sanctions must be documented, with documentation kept for six years.

- **Mitigation** (45 CFR §164.530(f)). A CE must mitigate, to the extent it can, any harmful effect that is known to the CE of a use or disclosure of PHI that was in violation of its policies and procedures.

- **Refraining from Intimidating or Retaliatory Acts** (45 CFR §164.530(g)). A CE may not intimidate, threaten, coerce, discriminate against, or take other retaliatory action against any individual who has filed a complaint against them.

- **Waiver of Rights** (45 CFR§164.530(h). A CE may not require individuals to waive its rights as a condition of treatment, payment, enrollment in a health plan, or eligibility for benefits.

- **Policies and Procedures** (45 CFR §164.530(i)). A CE must implement policies and procedures to protect PHI (taking into account the size and type of activities of the CE) to ensure compliance. When the law changes, the policies and procedures must be updated. Any changes made in the NPP must be reflected in updated policies and procedures. Likewise, if policies and procedures change, the NPP should be updated to reflect any changes. CEs should be sure the NPP includes the stipulation that the entity reserves its right to make changes to the NPP, so that changes can be in effect for PHI created or received prior to the effective date of the notice revision. Changes that are immaterial to the NPP can be made at any time.

- **Documentation** (45 CFR §164.530(j)). Policies and procedures must be maintained in written or electronic form and maintained for six years from the date of its creation or the date when it was last in effect, whichever is later.

- **Group Health Plans** (45 CFR §164.504(k)). Group health plans do not have to comply with some of these requirements, if certain conditions are met.

Summary

Under the regulations, PHI may be *used* (within a practice) and *disclosed* (outside of a practice) for TPO. There are specific situations where an authorization is not required for sharing PHI. These include releasing information to the individual, PHI used for TPO, for incidental uses and disclosures, and public health activities, and public interest and benefit activities, among others. Certain information may be released after the patient has had the opportunity to agree or object, to those involved in their care, if the CE reasonably infers consent, to assist notifications (e.g., death), and when an individual is incapacitated or in emergency circumstances. Without patient authorization, PHI may not be sold or used for marketing purposes or for genetic underwriting purposes.

A CE is required to verify that the person to whom they are releasing the PHI is authorized to receive it. Additionally, patients have the right to request certain restrictions on use or disclosure of their PHI. Personal representatives are treated in the same manner as if the patient requested the PHI. Patients may request restrictions on disclosing information to their health insurer if they pay out of pocket and other conditions are met. Disclosures to BAs require business associate agreements or other written contracts. Psychotherapy notes always require a written authorization. When releasing PHI for non-treatment purposes, the minimum necessary standard must be followed.

There are three types of health data: PHI, de-identified data, and a LDS. De-identified data and LDSs are often used for research, public health, or healthcare operations and do not require specific patient authorization, given certain criteria are met.

There are specific administrative requirements of the privacy regulations, which include designating a privacy official, training workforce on privacy of PHI, and other safeguards that must be in place to protect PHI. CEs must have a complaint process in place as well as a sanction policy for when privacy policies and procedures have been violated. Mitigation strategies must be used if PHI is compromised. The CE is expected to refrain from intimidating or retaliatory acts. Individual must not be expected to waive their rights in order to get treatment. Privacy policies and procedures must be developed, and documented (on paper or electronically).

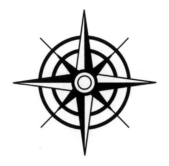

CHAPTER 5
Patient Rights and the Notice of Privacy Practices

Patient Rights under HIPAA and the HITECH Act

HIPAA granted patients specific privacy rights; in 2009 the Health Information Technology and Economic Clinical Health (HITECH) Act further increased patient rights. Covered Entities (CEs) may not require patients to waive any privacy rights as a condition for obtaining treatment, payment, or benefits eligibility. Specific patient privacy rights under HIPAA and HITECH include the following:

- The right to receive a Notice of Privacy Practices (NPP) outlining ways in which the CE may use or disclose their protected health information (PHI)

- The right to see and receive a copy of paper or Electronic Protected Health Information (EPHI) (at a reasonable, cost-based fee)

- The right to request changes or amend (e.g., correct errors) in medical records or add information they believe has been omitted

- The right to request confidential communications; a patient may request to communicate by alternative means or to an alternative location. For example, a patient may request that a message not be left at the home or that the bill is in a plain envelope

- The right to request special privacy protections of their PHI; for example, if the disclosure is for payment and healthcare operations and the patient has paid for the item or service in full, the CE may not disclose the PHI (unless legally required to do so)

- The right to view or receive a list of disclosures that have been made of the PHI, which is referred to as an Accounting of Disclosures (AOD)

- The right to choose a personal representative to act on their behalf

- The right to complain to the CE or Department of Health and Human Services (HHS) if a patient believes their privacy rights have been denied or violated

- The right to limit how PHI is used or disclosed for marketing and fundraising purposes or sale of their PHI.

Patient rights, and limitations to patient privacy set by the regulations, are communicated through a practice's own NPP. Business associates (BAs) are not required to create an NPP.

HIPAA DEMYSTIFIED

A Notice of Privacy Practices (NPP) communicates patients' rights to privacy, as well as limitations to privacy. Many practitioners use an NPP they have found online, often at their national professional association's website. A note of caution on a generic NPP: The Department of Health and Human Services specifically states that "The Notice must reflect any State law(s) that is more stringent than the Privacy Rule with respect to the use or disclosure of this information."[39] Be sure that you include more stringent state law in your NPP so your patients are correctly informed about their rights to privacy of their PHI, as well as legal limitations to those rights.

The Notice of Privacy Practices (45 CFR §164.520(a))

Patients receive an NPP to facilitate notice of the uses and disclosures of their PHI and the CEs legal duties with respect to PHI. The rights are communicated through a practice's NPP, which indicates specifically how the CE may use and disclose patient PHI.

The NPP must be made available at the first service date, barring emergencies. A good faith effort must be made to obtain the individual's written acknowledgement of the notice. If a patient or their representative is unwilling or unable to provide a signature, the CE should document the reason for failure to obtain the signature. The NPP does not need to be distributed each time a patient comes to your practice, but it must be made available upon request. It must also be prominently posted and needs to be made available at any website maintained by the practice or organization. A CE may e-mail the notice to a patient if the individual agrees to receive an electronic notice. If CEs perform various functions within the service delivery, variations of the NPP are allowed and should be as specific as possible.

As mentioned previously, when state laws are stricter, state laws should be followed (unless there is a federal preemption). Stricter state laws should be reflected in your NPP. In some cases, professional ethics codes will also designate a stricter course of action. There is also nothing that precludes your own set policies regarding confidentiality from being included in the NPP, given that they do not contradict state or federal regulations. A sample NPP for mental health practitioners is available in Appendix A.

The elements of the NPP include the following:

- **Header.** A statement as a header or otherwise prominently displayed that states: "THIS NOTICE DESCRIBES HOW MEDICAL INFORMATION ABOUT YOU MAY BE USED AND DISCLOSED AND HOW YOU CAN GET ACCESS TO THIS INFORMATION. PLEASE REVIEW IT CAREFULLY."

- **Uses and Disclosures.** A description of the types of disclosures that HIPAA allows without an authorization, including the following:

  o A description including at least one example of the types of disclosures that HIPAA permits the CE to make for treatment, payment, and healthcare operations (TPO)

  o A description of each of the other disclosures for which the CE is permitted or required to use or disclose PHI without the patient's authorization; these may include (a) to family members and others involved in the patient's healthcare unless the individual has objected; (b) to personal representatives; (c) to BAs or facility directories unless the patient objects; (d) as required by law (this includes child or elder abuse or domestic violence if state law allows); (e) to avert a serious threat or imminent harm to the patient or others; (f) for certain public health activities; (g) under certain conditions, for judicial or administrative proceedings; (h) for health oversight activities; (i) for judicial or administrative proceedings if certain conditions are met; (j) for specified law enforcement activities if certain conditions are met; (k) to the extent allowed by state workers compensation laws; (l) to coroners, medical examiners, or funeral directors; (m) for research purposes if certain conditions are met; and (n) for certain specialized government functions

  o A description of the types of uses and disclosures that require authorization, including psychotherapy notes, marketing, and sale of PHI; a specific statement is needed regarding marketing and fundraising, which states that the CE may contact the individual for these purposes, but that the individual has the right to opt out

  o A statement that other uses and disclosures not described in the NPP will be made only with the patient's written authorization (e.g., psychotherapy notes).

If the individual is incapacitated, it is an emergency situation, or if the patient is not available, CEs can use their professional judgment to determine if the disclosure is in the best interests of the patient. A CE may also rely on a patient's informal permission to disclose to a patient's family, relatives, friends, or others whom the patient identifies PHI relevant to that patient's involvement in the individual's care or payment of care. A CE may rely on informal permission to use and disclose PHI to notify family members or others responsible for the patient's care of their location, general condition, or death.

PHI may be disclosed if authorized by the patient to assist in disaster relief efforts.

- **Individual Rights.** Individual rights must be described, including the following:
  - o the right to request restrictions and uses or disclosures of their PHI for TPO
  - o the right to receive confidential communication by alternative means or at alternative locations (e.g., a patient may request email communication)
  - o the right to inspect and copy their PHI (with the exception of psychotherapy notes, depending upon state law)
  - o the right to amend their PHI
  - o the right to receive an accounting of disclosures of their PHI
  - o the right to request and receive a paper copy of the NPP
  - o a brief description of how the patient may exercise these rights (i.e., submitting a written request to your Privacy Official)
  - o authorization is required for most uses and disclosures of

psychotherapy notes

- o an authorization is required for use and disclosures of PHI for marketing purposes or disclosures that constitute sale of PHI

- o a statement that other uses and disclosures that are not described in the NPP will require an authorization

- o a statement that the individual may opt out of receiving fundraising communications

- o a statement that individuals who pay out of pocket in full for a healthcare item or service have the right to restrict disclosure of PHI to their health plan

- o a statement that they will be notified upon a breach of their PHI.

- o a statement must be made that indicates the patient who pays out of pocket in full for a healthcare item or service has the right to restrict disclosures of PHI to their health plan.

At least one example must be provided for when a CE is permitted to make disclosures for TPO.

- **Covered Entity Duties**. A statement of the CE's duties must be included, stating the CE will (a) maintain the privacy of the patient's PHI, (b) provide individuals with notice of its legal duties and privacy practices regarding their PHI, (c) notify them following a breach of their unsecured PHI, and (d) abide by the terms of the NPP and that the NPP will distribute any revised NPP to the patient. If the CE wishes to apply privacy practices changes to previously acquired PHI, the CE must include a statement to this effect (reserving the right to apply changes to all of the patient's PHI).

- **Complaints.** The following statements regarding complaints must be included: (a) the patient has a right to complain to the CE and to the secretary of HHS if they believe their privacy rights have been violated, (b) the patient will not be retaliated against for filing a complaint, and (c) the CE must provide the process for how to file a complaint with the CE (a CE is not required to detail how they can complain to HHS).

- **Contact Person.** The name or title of the contact person and telephone number must be provided for the person or office to contact for further information regarding their privacy rights.

- **Optional Information.** Check off boxes for patient approval or denial to provide appointment reminders, provide information on treatment alternatives, or marketing and fundraising solicitations as listed above may also be included.

- **Effective Date.** CEs must provide the effective date of the notice, which may not be earlier than the date of printing of the current NPP. The notice must include an effective date, and a CE is required to promptly revise and distribute its notice when it makes material changes to any of its privacy practices (within 60 days). HHS provides model notices on its website.

- **Revised Notice of Privacy Practices.** If HHS revises its NPP requirements (at the time of this writing the most recent was in 2013), a CE must revise the NPP, though the CE is not required to hand out a revised NPP to patients already in treatment. The revised NPP must be posted in a prominent location. You need to provide a revised NPP upon request. New patients need to receive the updated NPP with an effort on your part to obtain good faith acknowledgement of receipt. Again, if any use or disclosure is prohibited or limited by state law, the more stringent law should be reflected and described in the NPP.

- **Good Faith Effort of Written Acknowledgement.** Written acknowledgements of receipt of NPP or documentation of good faith efforts to obtain this acknowledgement should be documented and retained for at least six years. The acknowledgement may not be combined with other authorizations.

Additionally, the NPP must be in plain language. HHS provides examples of this in the model NPPs available at www.HHS.gov.[40] Examples of the plain language the HHS provides include the following verbiage:

"You have the right to:

- Get an electronic or paper copy of your medical record
- Ask us to correct your medical record
- Request confidential communications
- Ask us to limit what we use or share
- Get a list of those whom we've shared information with
- Get a copy of this privacy notice
- Choose someone to act for you
- File a complaint if you feel your rights have been violated."[41]

In addition, HHS notes that the patient has choices:

- "You may . . . [m]ake choices about how we share certain information (e.g. family, friends, in a disaster, and for fundraising)."
- "We never share your information unless you give us written permission for marketing purposes, sale of your information, or most sharing of psychotherapy notes."[42]

The NPP also notes uses and disclosures of PHI in the following manner:

- "We typically share information to treat you, run our organization, and bill for your services."
- "We may also share your information to help with public safety issues, do research, comply with the law, respond to organ and tissue donation request, work with a medical examiner or funeral director, address workers' compensation, law enforcement or other government requests, and respond to lawsuits and legal actions.
- "We may change the terms of this notice, which will be available upon request and on our website."[43]

It is the practitioner's responsibility to let the patient know about any breach that compromises patient privacy or security, follow the duties described in the NPP, and not share any other information beyond what is permitted in the NPP, unless permission is granted in writing.

Note that an NPP is not a static document: Revisions to the NPP are needed when there are material changes to patients' rights, changes to any uses and disclosures to their PHI, or any other changes dictated by HHS. Copies of all versions of the NPP and written acknowledgements of receipt of NPPs must be kept for six years from the date of the last effective date (be sure you have an effective date on the NPP).

The NPP can be provided electronically if the individual agrees to it. A paper copy of the NPP must be provided if you are aware that the email failed. If in an organized healthcare arrangement with other providers, there are additional requirements detailed on the HHS website.

HIPAA
DEMYSTIFIED

Your Notice of Privacy Practices (NPP) educates the patient about their rights and limitations to their confidentiality. It must be posted prominently where patients can see it, and it must be posted to your website. It need not be given to patients each time they come to your office (unless they request it). Covered entities are required to attempt to get acknowledgment of receipt of the NPP. Patients are not required to sign the acknowledgment, but if they do not, providers are still allowed to share protected health information as the HIPAA regulations allow. Providers should document patient refusal to sign the acknowledgment.

Request for Privacy Protections

Patients may request that they receive communications of PHI by alternate means or at alternate locations if the individual clearly states that the disclosure of all or part of their PHI could endanger them. A CE may require the privacy request be in writing and condition the provision to be a reasonable accommodation. A CE may not require the individual to explain the basis of the request as a condition of providing confidential services. Additionally, if a patient pays out of pocket, they may request that the CE not divulge information to an insurer.

Right to Request Privacy Protection for PHI

Patients have the right to request that a CE restrict use or disclosure of their PHI (45 CFR §164.522(a)) for the following reasons:

- for TPO
- from persons involved in their healthcare or payment for healthcare
- disclosures to notify family members or others about the individual's general condition, location, or death.

A CE must agree to an individual's request to restrict disclosure of PHI if the disclosures are for carrying out TPO and the individual has paid the CE for the service or item in full (unless legally prohibited).

Confidential Communications

A CE must permit individuals to request that they receive confidential communications of PHI by alternative means or at alternative locations (45 CFR §164.522(b)). The CE may require the individual to make the request in writing, condition the request upon establishing how payment will be handled, and specify an alternative address or method of contact.

Request for Amendments or Addendums to Records

Patients have the right to amendments or addendums to their medical records (not their psychotherapy notes (45 CFR §164.526(a)). The provider may consent or refuse the request for amendments or addendums, but must respond within 60 days to the request; one 30 day extension is allowed with written notice to the patient. Patients request may be made by email or web portal.

Patients have the right to appeal the CEs decision to deny access or amendment to the medical records. Unless state law allows access, if a patient requests access to psychotherapy notes, the request may be denied and is not appealable according to HIPAA regulations.

Request for an Accounting of Disclosures

Patients have a right to request an accounting of disclosures (AOD) for unauthorized disclosures of their medical records for the prior six years to the date that the patient is requesting record of disclosures (45 CFR §164.528(a)). CEs have 60 days to provide the AOD, with one 30 day extension with written notice to the individual. *Unauthorized* means that disclosures do not fall under the categories of TPO, HIPAA or state law reporting requirements, or a patient's authorization. At this time, you do not need to record disclosures for TPO (this may change in the future). The types of information that you do need to include in the AOD are:

- for public health purposes (e.g., communicable diseases)
- about victims of abuse, neglect, or domestic violence
- for health oversight activities (e.g., Medicare/Medicaid audits)
- for judicial or administrative proceedings (e.g., subpoenas and court orders)
- for law enforcement purposes (e.g., reporting of gunshot wounds)
- for coroners, medical examiners, or funeral directors (e.g., about deceased patients)

- for cadaveric organ, eye, or tissue donation and transplant purposes
- for human subject research that does not obtain a subject's authorization (e.g., research approved by an Institutional Review Board)
- to avert serious threat to health or safety
- to the Food and Drug Administration for purposes related to the quality, safety, or effectiveness of an FDA-regulated product or activity
- otherwise required or permitted by law (e.g., worker's compensation, state crime lab).

An AOD excludes the following information:

- for treatment (e.g., disclosures to other providers)
- for payment (e.g., third-party reimbursers)
- for healthcare operations (e.g., legal services, accreditation, licensing)
- for notification of or to persons involved in an individual's healthcare or payment for healthcare, for disaster relief, or for facility directories
- pursuant to an authorization (e.g., a signed authorization)
- that is part of a limited data set
- for national security or intelligence purposes (e.g., Homeland Security)
- to correctional institutions or law enforcement officials for certain purposes regarding inmates or individuals in lawful custody
- that is incidental to otherwise permitted or required uses or disclosures.

(H)IPAA DEMYSTIFIED

Talk to your IT person/company about how to run an Accounting of Disclosures (AOD) on electronic health records (EHRs). You may have to combine electronic information with paper if you keep paper records elsewhere. For those practices that use paper only, you may record disclosures on a ledger in the patient file. Disclosures to or by business associates also need to be included in the AOD. Most disclosures that are required to be in the AOD also require a release form, making it somewhat easier to track them.

If law enforcement officials or health oversight agencies indicate that disclosures would likely impede their activities, an AOD must be temporarily suspended. A CE must comply with written documentation from the official or agency that notes disclosure would impede their activities. Oral instructions from law enforcement officials or agencies are valid but must be documented; oral instructions are acceptable for 30 days (without further written statement).

The maximum disclosure accounting period is the six years immediately preceding the accounting request, except a CE is not obligated to account for any disclosure made before its Privacy Rule compliance date (April 14, 2003). Patients also have a right to an AOD from your BAs.

There are several options for tracking disclosures. Within EHRs a tracking system should be available, sorting by individual and date. Another option is to keep a manual log of disclosures. Lastly, an authorization form may be used as a mechanism for tracking (listing the reason for the disclosure), but not all releases of PHI will be included via authorization forms and will need to be augmented by other records. Your specific policies and procedures should include this process.

Additional Requirements Regarding the NPP

Dissemination of the NPP requires several additional requirements:

- There must be a "good faith effort" to obtain written acknowledgement of the receipt of the NPP. If unable to do so, it should be documented that an attempt was made, and the reason why the acknowledgement could not be obtained should also be documented.

- The NPP must be provided no later than the first date of service including any electronic contact/delivery.

- If there is an emergency situation that prevented the dispersing of the NPP, the notice must be provided in a reasonable time period after the emergency is managed.

- If a website is maintained, the NPP must also be "prominently" posted on the website.

- The notice must be posted in a clear and prominent location at the point of service.

- A paper copy of the NPP must be available for patients.

- The NPP must be available upon request. If the NPP is revised, it must be available upon request on or after the effective date of the revision.[44]

Summary

When dealing with PHI, "use" refers to sharing of PHI internal to an organization, while "disclosure" refers to sharing of PHI outside of an organization. PHI may be freely shared for TPO, with few exceptions; psychotherapy notes may not be released without an authorization. In an emergency, information can be revealed unless the provider knows from a previous conversation that the patient does not want information released to a certain person.

When releasing information for non-TPO purposes, the minimum necessary standard should be followed. Patients have the right to request restrictions to release of their PHI. De-identified data may be released without an authorization. De-identification occurs when the 18 PHI identifiers are removed, or when a statistician has ruled that there is negligible risk to link the PHI to the individual.

Patients have the right to an AOD, which reveals disclosures made for non-TPO purposes, including verbal disclosures. All privacy rights and limitations to a patient's privacy rights must be detailed in an organization's NPP.

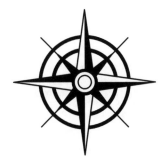

CHAPTER 6
HIPAA and Treatment Records

The privacy regulations outline two types of records: the designated record set (DRS) and the legal health record (LHR). Both the DRS and the LHR will be introduced in this chapter. Additionally, treatment record information such as record retention, access to treatment records, denials, response time, and record fees will be addressed. As with all of your compliance efforts, your state law must also be examined to understand your exact requirements regarding treatment records. Some states include mental health records in their medical records statutes, while others have separate regulations for mental health records.

Designated Record Set (45 CFR §164.524)

To facilitate disclosure of Protected Health Information (PHI), covered entities (CEs) need to establish the DRS, which is information that a patient has the right to access and includes your medical and billing records. It is any information an organization uses to inform treatment decisions (sans psychotherapy notes). *Record* means any item, collection, or grouping of information that includes PHI and is maintained, collected, used, or disseminated by or for a CE (45 CFR §164.501). Specifically, the

DRS is defined by the Department of Health and Human Services (HHS) as a group of records maintained that include:

- medical and billing records
- any information used in whole or in part by or for the healthcare plan or provider that is used to make treatment decisions about individuals
- a health plan's enrollment, payment, claims adjudication, and case or medical management record systems maintained for or by a health plan.

The DRS is important particularly in regards to electronic health records (EHRs) where much information is kept. Patients are not privy to all the information a CE collects; thus, the DRS defines what information may be accessed. Patients may also petition to amend portions of their DRS, but not the LHR.

Legal Health Record (45 CFR §164.501)

Practices should establish guidelines for what is to be included in the LHR. This record identifies what information constitutes your business record for evidentiary purposes. For example, these records that support treatment decisions or support reimbursement requests from third-party payers should be included in the DRS.

Your practice or organization should determine a records retention policy so that the DRS and LHR are clearly defined. Policies and procedures around these records should be established with regard to state law and with consultation with your attorney. Policies and procedures should be in place that determine how records requests from external sources will be handled (state law may address this). The LHR clarifies what information is to be used for evidentiary purposes; the DRS clarifies what information patients have access to.

In the past, this distinction was not necessary, but with the advent of EHRs, designation was needed to clarify to what information patients had access within the EHR.

⊕IPAA
DEMYSTIFIED

You will want to decide what you consider your designated record set as to what information patients may access. Additionally, you will want to decide what is included in your legal health record for evidentiary purposes. These definitions should be included in your policies and procedures.

Records Retention

Under HIPAA regulations, there are no medical or mental health record requirements; instead state statutes on record retention should be followed. Additionally, specific programs may have specific records retention policies. For example, Medicare Advantage plans and their contracted providers must retain medical records, financial records, and source reports for a period of 10 years. Of all applicable regulations, the most stringent (greater retention time) should be followed.

⊕IPAA
DEMYSTIFIED

HIPAA defers to state law with regard to how long practitioners should keep medical/mental health records. However, documentation related to HIPAA policies and procedures, and any actions taken in response to those procedures (e.g., workforce training materials), must be kept for six years.

Request for Access to Patient Records (45 CFR §164.524)

Patients have the right to review or obtain copies of their medical records that are maintained in their DRS (see Chapter 5). The medical records exclude psychotherapy notes, but include other counseling information.

Requests for record access must be responded to within 30 days of the request. A 30-day extension is allowed, but you must provide the patient with written notice stating the reason for the delay and the expected delivery date. This applies to both paper and electronic records. State law may require shorter time periods for responding to requests, and if so, the shorter time period should be followed.

Under HIPAA regulations, patients may not have access to their psychotherapy notes; individuals and their personal representatives may access their other mental health/medical records. Personal representatives are those legally authorized to act on behalf of the individual regarding healthcare issues such as healthcare powers of attorney or those with parental rights of minors. HIPAA does not designate rights of minors, but defers to state law for clarification of both minor status (i.e. age of consent) and parental rights to mental health information. The CE should verify the identity of the person requesting access (orally or in writing). Again, patients, or their representatives, do not have access to psychotherapy notes unless state law grants it.

CEs must provide access to a patient's PHI in the form of patient requests (i.e., electronic or paper). A summary of the information may be provided instead, if the individual agrees to the alternate format and fees. Patients may ask for an electronic copy of their records; it may be downloaded to a compact disk or USB drive. For cyber security, it is recommended the CE provide the compact disk or USB themselves. If an electronic copy of PHI is not available, paper must be provided. If reasonable safeguards are in place, records may be emailed at the patient's request.

If patients request that their PHI be sent to a third party (outside of treatment, payment, and healthcare operations purposes (TPO)) a written, signed authorization is needed. The authorization needs to designate what records they wish released, to whom they are to be released, and where the records are to be sent.

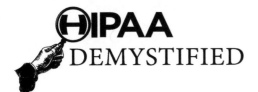

Patients (or their personal representatives) may have access to their medical/mental health records. However, they may not have access to psychotherapy notes as defined by the regulations; this denial is not appealable. Any state law, that gives the patient more access to their records, would supersede HIPAA regulations.

Grounds for Denial to Access of Patient Records
(45 CFR §164.524(b)(2)(i))

There are a few instances where CEs are allowed to deny access to records. These include, first and foremost, psychotherapy notes. This is not appealable. Other instances of denials that are not appealable include information compiled for legal proceedings, certain information held by clinical laboratories, certain requests made by correctional institutions, certain information obtained during research, or denials permitted by the Privacy Act of 1974. Access to PHI that was obtained from someone other than a healthcare practitioner under a promise of confidentiality may be denied when access would likely reveal the source of the information.

Other grounds for denial that the patient may appeal include disclosures that would cause endangerment to the patient or another individual. Denials must be written with a description of the basis for the denial and, if it is an appealable request, a statement of the individual's right to have the decision reviewed with instructions on how to request a review.

A statement of how to file complaints regarding the denial must also be provided. Should the individual make the request electronically, a denial may also be made electronically. Denials must be made within 30 days. For any extensions on the part of the CE, the individual must be provided with a written notice explaining the reason for the delay. Only one such 30 day extension is allowed.

Fees (45 CFR §164.524)

You may charge a reasonable cost-based fee for providing a copy of requested records. Cost-based includes labor, supplies, postage, or the cost of preparing a summary of PHI if the individual has agreed to a summary. Importantly, state law may set a fee or limitation of what may be reimbursed; the smaller fee applies. HIPAA is silent on what a CE may charge outside entities for copies of records, providers are encouraged to consult state law for guidance on fees for outside entities (entities other than the patient or their personal representative).

Summary

CEs need to be able to identify two types of record sets. The first is the DRS, to which patients have access. The second is the LHR, which is used to support treatment decisions or support reimbursement requests from third-party payers, and used for evidentiary purposes. HIPAA does not require that treatment records be retained for any particular length of time, though state law or other government program laws may have specifications on record retention. HIPAA does not designate parental access to treatment information of minors, but instead defers to state law. In response to record requests, a cost-based fee may be assessed.

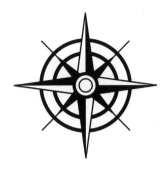

CHAPTER 7

An Introduction to the Security Requirements

One reason the HIPAA compliance can seem overwhelming is that there are 54 required or addressable HIPAA standards and implementation specifications in the security regulations[46] alone. These requirements are divided into three safeguard areas: administrative, physical, and technical. We will explore these three safeguard areas in detail in the following chapters. A summary of the safeguards is available in Tables 7.1, 7.2, and 7.3.

All of the standards and implementation specifications within the safeguards must be evaluated in your practice. Standards are regulations set by HIPAA to ensure appropriate administrative, physical, and technical safeguards to ensure the confidentiality, integrity, and availability of Electronic Protected Health Information (EPHI). Implementation specifications are a more detailed description of the method or approach covered entities (CEs) can use to meet a particular standard.

While all HIPAA standards are required, implementation specifications can be required or addressable. *Required* means that the implementation specifications are to be implemented as stated in the regulation. *Addressable* means that you have more flexibility in deciding how to meet the specification. With addressable specifications, the CE must determine how to implement the specification based on what is reasonable and appropriate. What does "reasonable and appropriate" mean? A CE may consider: (1) the size, complexity, and capabilities of an organization; (2) the costs of the security measures; (3) the organization's current technical infrastructure, hardware, and software; and (4) the likelihood that the risks will occur and the seriousness of the impact on the organization's EPHI and business operations. Therefore, smaller practices have more leeway in scaling the addressable requirements to fit their needs. It is important to remember that no standard or implementation specification is optional; all must be addressed in your practice.

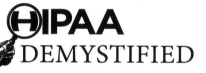

All of the 54 HIPAA security standards and implementation specifications must be evaluated and addressed in your practice. HIPAA implementation specifications are either *required* or *addressable*. Required means you must implement the specification as stated. Addressable means that you may take into account the resources of your practice when evaluating how to implement the specification. Addressable does not mean optional! In the unlikely event you believe that an addressable implementation specification does not apply to you, you must document your reason for not adopting the specification.

Administrative Safeguards

By far the largest areas of safeguards in your HIPAA compliance, administrative safeguards, consist of administrative actions and policies and procedures to manage the selection, development, and implementation of security measures to protect EPHI. It also includes measures to manage the CE's workforce in efforts to maintain security of PHI.[47]

Standard	Implementation Specification
Security Management Process 45 CFR §164.308(a)(1)	• Risk Analysis (R) 45 CFR §164.308(a)(1)(ii)(A) • Risk Management (R) 45 CFR §164.308(a)(1)(ii)(B) • Sanction Policy (R) 45 CFR §164.308(a)(1)(ii)(C) • Information System Activity Review (R) 45 CFR §164.308(a)(1)(ii)(D)
Assigned Security Responsibility 45 CFR §164.308(a)(2)	• Required Standard
Workforce Security 45 CFR §164.308(a)(3)	• Authorization and/or Supervision (A) 45 CFR §164.308(a)(3) • Workforce Clearance Procedure (A) 45 CFR §164.308(a)(3)(ii)(B) • Termination Procedures (A) 45 CFR §164.308(a)(3)(ii)(C)
Information Access Management 45 CFR §164.308(a)(4)	• Isolating Healthcare Clearinghouse Functions (R) 45 CFR §164.308(a)(4)(ii)(A) • Access authorization (A) 45 CFR §164.308(a)(4)(ii)(B) • Access establishment and modification (A) 45 CFR §164.308(a)(4)(ii)(C)
Security Awareness Training 45 CFR §164.308(a)(5)	• Security Reminders (A) 45 CFR §164.308(a)(5)(ii)(A) • Protection from Malicious Software (A) 45 CFR §164.308(a)(5)(ii)(B) • Log-in Monitoring (A) 45 CFR §164.308(a)(5)(ii)(C) • Password Management (A) 45 CFR §164.308(a)(5)(ii)(D)

Standard	Implementation Specification
Security Incident Procedures 45 CFR §164.308(a)(6)	• Response and Reporting (R) 45 CFR §164.308(a)(6)(ii)
Contingency Plan 45 CFR §164.308(a)(7)	• Data Backup Plan (R) 45 CFR §164.308(a)(7)(ii)(A) • Disaster Recovery Plan (R) 45 CFR §164.308(a)(7)(ii)(B) • Emergency Mode Operation Plan (R) 45 CFR §164.308(a)(7)(ii)(C) • Testing and Revision Procedure (A) 45 CFR §164.308(a)(7)(ii)(D) • Applications and Data Criticality Analysis (A) 45 CFR §164.308(a)(7)(ii)(E)
Business Associate Contracts and Other Arrangements 45 CFR §164.308(b)(1)	• Written contracts or other arrangement (R) 45 CFR §164.308(b)(4)

Table 7.1. Administrative safeguards (R = Required; A = Addressable)

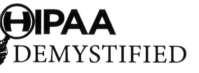

It is likely that you already have several administrative safeguards in place. Your practice may have an employee sanction policy, termination policy, and written contracts with outside service providers. You need to address (and document) your handling of the Administrative Safeguards.

Physical Safeguards

Physical safeguards are the physical measures, policies, and procedures to protect your electronic information systems related to your buildings and equipment. These measures help to ensure that the EPHI in your building and housed within your equipment is safe from natural and environmental hazards and unauthorized intrusion. All physical access to EPHI must be considered, including any that extends beyond your actual office, including workforce member's homes or other physical locations where EPHI[48] can be accessed.

Facility Access Controls 45 CFR §164.310(a)(1)	• Contingency Operations (A) 45 CFR §164.310(a)(2)(i) • Facility Security Plan (A) 45 CFR §164. 310(a)(2)(ii) • Access Control and Validation Procedures (A) 45 CFR §164.310(a)(2)(iii) • Maintenance Records (A) 45 CFR §164.310(a)(2)(iv)
Workstation Use 45 CFR §164.310(b)	• Required Standard
Device and Media Controls 45 CFR §164.310(d)(1)	• Disposal (R) 45 CFR §164.310(d)(2)(i) • Media Re-use (R) 45 CFR §164.310(d)(2)(ii) • Accountability (A) 45 CFR §164.310(d)(2)(iii) • Data Backup and Storage (A) 45 CFR §164.310(d)(2)(iv)

Table 7.2. Physical safeguards (R = Required; A = Addressable)

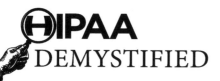

Your practice likely has various physical safeguards already in place. These include building security measures such as alarm systems, visitor policies, and fire protection mechanisms. You also likely already have workstation policies regarding who is allowed past your reception desk, rules about office security, and so on. Typically practices backup their electronic patient data. These are all examples of physical safeguards.

Technical Safeguards

Technical safeguards are the technology, and the policies and procedures for the use and control of technology that protect EPHI.[49] No specific types or rules of technology are identified or required. This includes policies and procedures that outline how the workforce is to manage and protect the technology used to create, receive, maintain, or transmit EPHI.

Access Control
45 CFR §164.312(a)(1)
	• Unique User Identification (R)
	  45 CFR §164.312(a)(2)(i)
	• Emergency Access Procedure (R)
	  45 CFR §164.312(a)(2)(ii)
	• Automatic Logoff (A)
	  45 CFR §164.312(a)(2)(iii)
	• Encryption and Decryption (A)
	  45 CFR §164.312(a)(2)(iv)

Audit Controls 45 CFR §164.312(b)	• Required Standard
Integrity 45 CFR §164.312(c)(1)	• Mechanism to Authenticate EPHI (A) 45 CFR §164.312(c)(2)

Person or Entity Authentication 45 CFR §164.312(d)	• Required Standard

Transmission Security
45 CFR §164.312(e)(1)
	• Integrity Controls (A)
	  45 CFR §164.312(e)(2)(i)
	• Encryption (A)
	  45 CFR §164.312(e)(2)(ii)

Table 7.3. Technical safeguards (R = Required; A = Addressable)

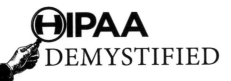

HIPAA
DEMYSTIFIED

Technical safeguards may include mechanisms that log off your computers after a predetermined period of time, with each workforce member having their own credentials to log in to your system. Be sure to address each standard and implementation specification (and document).

Summary

HIPAA security compliance involves standards and implementation specifications, some of which are required and some of which are addressable, housed within administrative, physical, or technical safeguards. All must be considered and evaluated within your practice. Required standards and implementation specifications must be followed as stated in the regulations. Addressable implementation specifications are scalable: you can consider the specific needs of your organization based on evaluating the size, complexity, capabilities, costs, and current infrastructure when evaluating risks to your EPHI.

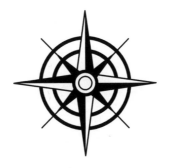

CHAPTER 8
Security Risk Assessment

The HIPAA Security Rule requires organizations to implement a security management process to identify and analyze risks to Electronic Protected Health Information (EPHI), and subsequently implement security measures to remediate those risks. Generally, this includes evaluating threats to your patient EPHI, evaluating the adequacy of existing privacy and security measures, evaluating potential future threats, and barriers to adoption.[50] The role of the security risk assessment (SRA) is crucial to establishing and maintaining HIPAA compliance. The SRA helps to ensure the confidentiality, integrity, availability[51] of EPHI. Risk management is not a static process; you must continually monitor and evaluate your practice to ensure security of your practice's PHI. The U.S. Department of Health and Human Services (HHS) takes a "media neutral" policy toward PHI, meaning that any data must be protected, whether it is in electronic, paper, or oral format. While not technically required, note that in the privacy regulations, administrative, physical and technical safeguards are also required to protect paper PHI (45 CFR 164.530(c)). The SRA can be adapted for PHI in addition to EPHI.

In this chapter we will explore how to conduct the SRA from inventory of EPHI sources, to evaluating specific risks, evaluating risk mitigation strategies you already have in place, and culminating in understanding the risk remediation plan. The role of your business associates in your SRA will also be discussed.

Risk Analysis and Risk Management (45 CFR §164.308(a)(1)(ii)(A), (Required); (45 CFR §164.308(a)(1)(ii)(B)), (Required))

The SRA includes both risk analysis and risk management. Risk analysis requires you to conduct an accurate and thorough assessment of potential threats and vulnerabilities to the confidentiality, integrity, and availability, of your PHI. The SRA should address how EPHI is generated, accessed, transmitted, and stored. Risk management requires you to implement security measures sufficient to reduce vulnerabilities to a "reasonable and appropriate" level. While reasonable and appropriate is rather nebulous, it is not assumed that covered entities (CEs) or business associates (BAs) will never have any breach of PHI. You are expected, however, to minimize that risk through good policies, procedures, and practices. Ultimately, you will generate security policies and procedures with the goal of preventing, detecting, containing, and correcting security violations using ongoing vulnerability or threat analyses. Policies and procedures for risk analysis and risk management will vary according to the degree to which you use electronic storage and transmit of EPHI in your practice.

Security Risk Assessment Procedure

The SRA can be a lengthy process; at times it can feel daunting. Help for this process is available from HHS[52] and the National Institute for Standards and Technology;[53] privacy requirements may be assessed in the same manner.

The process for an SRA includes several steps from inventory, evaluating risks, determining the likelihood of threats, remediating those threats, documenting, and monitoring the effectiveness of the strategies put in place to address the risk.

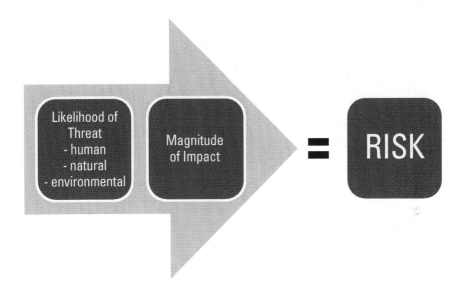

Figure 8.1. Risk is a function of threat x magnitude of impact of the threat

A vulnerability is a potential flaw or weakness in your security procedures (both technical and non-technical), which increases the likelihood that a threat will occur. The goal of the risk analysis is to decrease vulnerabilities by increasing security, maintaining, or developing good policies and procedures to protect your PHI/EPHI, as well as training the workforce on those policies and procedures. Risk includes evaluating the impact of a threat, be it of human, natural or environmental origin, and determining the magnitude of impact of that threat should it come to fruition.

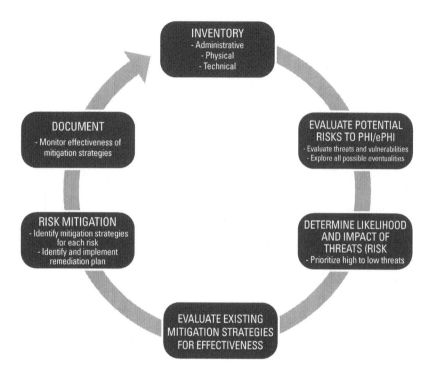

Figure 8.2. Security risk assessment procedure[54,55,56]

Inventory

The first step of the SRA is to take inventory. Inventory includes surveying physical and technical inventory. Inventory also includes facilities and processes where data is created, stored, received, maintained, or transmitted. This includes physical inventory, such as your office building, your office, specific rooms, and specific departments. It also includes technical inventory, such as your computers, workstations, portable data devices, network devices, hardware, software, storage media (e.g., hard drives, USBs, CDs), and telecommunications devices. Refer to figure 8.3 for an example of items you may need to include in your technical inventory. Remote access to EPHI should also be inventoried. A personnel inventory of who has access to data is important, with their prescribed access documented.

⊕IPAA
DEMYSTIFIED

Within the security risk assessment, inventory consists of your practice's property, facilities, telecommunications, hardware, software, and people who have access to PHI/EPHI. Don't forget portable media devices such as phones and laptops.

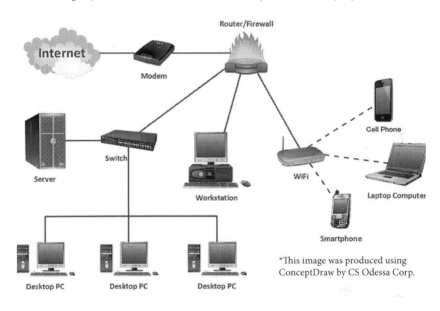

Figure 8.3. Potential technical inventory for SRA

Evaluating Potential Risks to PHI/EPHI

You must evaluate vulnerabilities and threats of the technical and nontechnical aspects of your practice; vulnerabilities are inherent weaknesses or absences of a safeguard.[57] Vulnerabilities include all of the flaws and weaknesses in your technical and nontechnical security procedures. These vulnerabilities include nature (e.g., tornadoes, hurricanes, lightning, earthquakes), human (e.g., carelessness, errors, unauthorized access, identity theft, tampering, hacking, malicious code, and theft of equipment by internal workforce members), or environmental (e.g., power outage, break in a network cable, plumbing problem).[58] Threat is the likelihood that these will occur or be triggered. It is recommended that you explore all "reasonably anticipated" threats.[59] Reasonably anticipated are those threats that we would expect of an ordinary person to consider in the same or similar circumstances based on geographic location, statistics, past experiences, and industry trends.[60] For example, if your office is in a flood plain, most people would reasonably anticipate flooding as a threat. Threats can target vulnerabilities when data is at rest, while in use, or while in transit.[61] Common threats to EPHI that could be considered "reasonably anticipated" include (1) unauthorized disclosure, such as when PHI is breached; (2) corruption, such as accidental modification to data; (3) denial of service where resources are made unavailable; and (4) the inability to prove the source of an attack, such as when someone performs an unauthorized activity using a shared account.[62]

HIPAA DEMYSTIFIED

You must evaluate all of the potential flaws and weaknesses in your technical and nontechnical security procedures (vulnerabilities), and the likelihood that they may occur (threat). The areas with the highest risk should be addressed first. Risks may be evaluated using your current policies and procedures, interviewing key players, brainstorming eventualities, and reviewing existing risk mitigation strategies.

Determining Likelihood and Impact of Threats (Risk Analysis)

During your risk analysis, threats must be prioritized from high to low on both likelihood of their occurrence, as well as impact of the threat to patients this allows you to make well-informed decisions about which risks need to be addressed and the degree to which it is appropriate to mitigate the risks.[63] There are two common ways to determine the risk that events may affect your practice. The first is a qualitative risk analysis, which is examining the likelihood of threat for your inventory items, as well as the effect or severity of the threat should it come to pass. The threats can be divided into categories of high, moderate, and low, but you may also expand the detail of the categories for more detailed analysis. Additionally, quantitative analysis is available where dollar amounts are given to categories of threat. This is difficult to do, especially in the healthcare fields, so most providers perform qualitative analyses.

Impact of Threat (Severity)	Likelihood of Threat		
	HIGH	MODERATE	LOW
HIGH	HIGH	HIGH	MODERATE
MODERATE	MODERATE	MODERATE	LOW
LOW	MODERATE	LOW	LOW

Table 8.1. Qualitative risk analysis matrix illustrative of impact and likelihood of treat[64]

Another option for risk analysis is a model that combines qualitative and quantitative methods. In this model, numbers are assigned to the threat and potential effect.

LIKELIHOOD OF THREAT			
	HIGH (100)	MODERATE (50)	LOW (10)
HIGH (1.0)	High $100 \times 1.0 = 100$	Moderate $50 \times 1.0 = 50$	Moderate $10 \times 1.0 = 10$
MODERATE (.5)	Moderate $100 \times .5 = 50$	Moderate $50 \times .5 = 25$	Low $10 \times .5 = 5$
LOW (.1)	Moderate $100 \times .1 = 10$	Low $50 \times .1 = 5$	Low $10 \times .1 = 1$

(Left vertical axis label: Impact of Threat (Magnitude))

Note: High range=75 to 100; Medium range=26 to 74; Low range=1 to 25

Table 8.2. Qualitative and semi-quantitative risk analysis[65]

Each safeguard (administrative, physical, and technical) must be addressed in detail. The likelihood of the threat and the risk level is to be determined (e.g., low, medium, or high) and remediation planned, according to the outcome of your analysis.

Threat	Vulnerability	Likelihood Rating	Impact Rating	Risk Rating
Inappropriate use or disclosure of PHI	45 CFR §164.08 (a)(3)(ii)(B) Workforce Clearance: Office staff has complete access to mental health records.	HIGH	High: Mental health information is sensitive PHI, which could lead to breach of privacy for patients.	HIGH

Threat	Vulnerability	Likelihood Rating	Impact Rating	Risk Rating
Sharing of passwords	45 CFR §164.308(a)(5)(ii)(D) No policy exists to discourage sharing of passwords among the workforce.	Medium	Medium: Inappropriate access of mental health information in violation of the "minimum necessary."	Medium

Table 8.3. Examples of items that may be included in your risk analysis

Evaluating Existing Mitigation Strategies for Effectiveness

After the initial risk analysis is performed, you will want to evaluate your present controls or mitigation strategies with the likelihood and severity of the threat in mind. These are your existing policies, procedures, and practices. Risk mitigation strategies can include improvements in physical security, technical security, and security awareness and training.

Risk Mitigation

Risk mitigation strategies will be assigned according to the level the threat poses to the confidentiality, integrity, availability, or accountability of your PHI/EPHI based on our risk analysis and review of existing mitigation strategies. Mitigation strategies must be established for each risk, starting with those items that have the highest level of risk. The goal is to decrease the likelihood or effect of the threat being acted upon. Typically, remediation is conducted first for high-risk items. Mitigation strategies should include the risk score, the threat, an action plan to mitigate the risk, an assignee(s) who is responsible for implementing the action plan, and a target date (see Table 8.4).

Risk Score	Threat	Action Plan	Assignee	Target Date
High	45 CFR §164.308(a)(3)(ii)(B) Workforce Clearance: Implement procedures to determine that the access of a workforce member to EPHI is appropriate.	Implement policies and procedures to base access to EPHI by workforce roles.	Jane Brown	1/31/16
Medium	45 CFR §164.308(a)(5)(ii)(D) Password Management: Implement procedures for creating, changing, and safeguarding passwords.	Implement policies and procedures to manage security of passwords.	John White	1/31/16

Table 8.4. Risk mitigation plan

There are four ways to address the risks. For some risks, you may want to simply accept the risk. For example, if your practice is in a higher crime area, you may wish to install security features beyond door locks, such as security cameras or alarm systems. However, these efforts may be cost prohibitive to your practice so you accept the risk and do nothing other than secure door locks. You may choose to avoid the risk; for example you may choose to relocate your practice into a less crime-ridden neighborhood. You may choose to transfer the risk by shifting responsibility or liability to another party. For instance, you move your practice into an office where the landlord manages security measures for the entire building, providing measures to decrease security risks. The last option is to mitigate the risk by using strict security policies and procedures, instructing the workforce to monitor people who show up without an appointment, establish clear evening lock-up instructions, and so on.[66,67]

Documenting and Monitoring Effectiveness of Mitigation Strategies

Once mitigation strategies have been identified, to remediate the risk, parties who are responsible for executing the mitigation strategy, and target dates must be established. Mitigation efforts should be documented. All mental health professionals know the dictate: "If you didn't document, it didn't happen." Additionally, it is wise to document temporary acceptance of a risk while you work on remediating it.[68]

Threat environments are constantly changing so monitoring your controls is essential to your risk management. Additionally, security gaps should be identified, monitored, and included in the risk analysis process as needed. Regular, scheduled reevaluation is needed. Reevaluation may also be triggered by a change in legal or regulatory requirements, a change in security policy, and so on.[69]

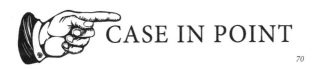 CASE IN POINT

[70]

Cancer Care Group, P.C., was fined $750,000 for not having completed a security risk analysis. The group had a laptop bag stolen from an employee's car, which contained unencrypted protected health information, including social security numbers, insurance information, and patient clinical information of 55,000 patients. The Office for Civil Rights (OCR) found that Cancer Care had not conducted a security risk assessment, nor did they have in place written policies specific to removal of hardware or electronic media containing electronic protected health information into and out of its facilities, even though it was a common occurrence, contributing to the breach. OCR maintained had Cancer Care had these policies and procedures, this type of breach may have been prevented.

Due Diligence on Business Associates

As part of your SRA, you also need to assess BAs for their compliance with the regulations. Areas on which to focus during this portion of your assessment should include areas that the most recent HIPAA audits include. Typically these involve evaluating whether your BAs have updated policies and procedures that are accessible, whether they have conducted recent, relevant HIPAA training with their workforce, whether or not the BAs themselves have conducted their own SRA, and established a remediation plan, where they are addressing risks to PHI/EPHI. Your practice must evidence ongoing assessment of risks and threats to PHI. BAs are responsible for evaluating their subcontractors for compliance with the regulations.

Summary

SRAs are the foundation of any security plan. The end goal of an SRA is a remediation plan to address any identified security gaps, conduct training with appropriate personnel on the new policies and procedures, and document changes in policies and procedures. CEs need to demonstrate that the remediation plan has been created and accepted, and that the organization is making meaningful progress through the plan. SRAs must be done at least annually, but also periodically when you have changes in your practice operations or workforce. You should have an integrated program of policies and procedures, organizational accountability, and training, potentially including a monthly or quarterly test schedule to scan for system vulnerabilities.

HHS provides a template for an SRA, and NIST provides guidelines for risk management (see Appendix B: Sources of Help). Because you are responsible and liable for breaches by your BAs, you also need to ensure that your BAs are safeguarding your PHI. BAs, however, are responsible for evaluating the compliance of their subcontractors.

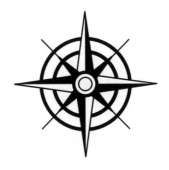

CHAPTER 9
Administrative Safeguards

Administrative safeguards are all administrative actions and policies and procedures in place to manage the selection, development, implementation, and maintenance of measures to protect Electronic Protected Health Information (EPHI), as well as to ensure that the covered entities' workforce conducts itself in a manner conducive to protecting the security of EPHI. A covered entity (CE) must have an overall security management process, which requires a CE to detect and correct security breaches (45 CFR §164.308(a)(1)), and each CE is required to assign a chief security official (45 CFR §164.308(a)(2)). A CE must also provide for workforce security, (45 CFR §164.308), allowing for appropriate access to EPHI, as well as having safeguards in place about inappropriate access, through information access management (45 CFR §164.308(a)(4)(i)) policies and procedures. Security awareness and training (45 CFR §164.308(a) (5)) must occur, and security incident procedures (45 CFR §164.308(a)(6) (ii)) need to be in place, and contingency plans (45 CFR 164.308(a)(7)(i)) established. To maintain security of EPHI, evaluation of the administrative safeguards (45 CFR §164.308(a)(8)) must occur on a regular basis. Lastly, business associate (BA) contracts, or other written arrangements (45 CFR §164.308(b)(1)), are required to protect EPHI that is handled by those your practice contracts with who must have access to EPHI to do their job.

What follows are questions adapted in part from the U.S. Department of Health and Human Services (HHS) Security Risk Assessment (SRA)[71], a joint effort of the Department of Health and Human Services (HHS) Office of the National Coordinator for Health Information Technology and Office for Civil Rights (OCR), as well as the National Institute of Standards and Technology (NIST) special publication 800-30 Guide for Conducting Risk Assessments[72] with further explanation to "demystify" the safeguards.

———●———

***Workforce** refers to employees, volunteers, trainees, and other persons whose conduct, in the performance of work for a CE, is under the direct control of such entity, whether or not they are paid by the covered entity (45 CFR §160.103).*

———●———

Security Management Process

✪ **Does your organization have documented policies and procedures for assessing and managing risk to it's EPHI? Are the policies and procedures periodically reviewed and updated as necessary?**

Security Management Process (45 CFR §164.308(a)(1)), (Required Standard). This standard requires CEs to "Implement policies and procedures to prevent, detect, contain and correct security violations." The purpose of this standard is to establish the administrative processes and procedures that a CE will use to implement the security program in its environment. Policies and procedures must be documented.

(H)IPAA
DEMYSTIFIED

You must have policies and procedures regarding all facets of your electronic protected health information and keep them updated as your practice makes changes in operations. They must also be available to relevant workforce members. Be sure to date all of your policies and procedures, both for your own reference, and in the event of an audit.

Risk Analysis

✪ **Have you performed an SRA? Have you conducted a risk assessment of potential risks and vulnerabilities to your protected health information? Is your risk assessment periodically reviewed? Have you categorized your EPHI in your IT system considering the potential effect to your practice or operations?**

Risk Analysis (45 CFR §164.308(a)(1)(ii)(A)), (Required). As discussed in chapter 8, you are required to develop, document, and implement policies and procedures for assessing and managing risk to your EPHI. Your organization must perform a risk analysis (security risk analysis) to evaluate the confidentiality, availability, and integrity of your organization's data. One tool is the OCR Division of Health Information Privacy (http://www.healthit.gov/providers-professionals/security-risk-assessment-tool).

Risk analysis includes evaluation of all of the EPHI flowing throughout your organization, identifies a process for evaluating potential security risks, determines the probability of the occurrence of the risks, and weighs the magnitude of the risk.[73] HHS does not designate a method or best practice to complete an SRA. You are to look for vulnerabilities and threats to your EPHI.

As mentioned in chapter 8, a CE must estimate risk by evaluating both the likelihood and potential impact of the threat.

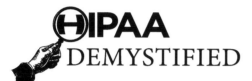

You must do an security risk assessment for your practice(s) to assess risk of security violations to patient protected health information and regularly review it. You are also required to evaluate the compliance of your business associates with having done their own security risk assessment(s).

Risk Management

✪ **Have you implemented (and documented) a risk remediation plan after you have performed your SRA?**

Risk Management (45 CFR §164.308(a)(1)(ii)(B)), (Required). An organization must make decisions about how to address security risks and vulnerabilities to their EPHI. You must remediate risks you identified in your SRA to a "reasonable and appropriate" level. You must implement and document, risk remediation—corrective policies and procedures that address the risks found in the SRA and prevent against impermissible use and disclosure of EPHI. Appropriate workforce should be assigned remediation tasks. These policies and procedures should be kept in mind when purchases of new hardware and software are made.

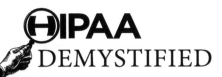

HIPAA DEMYSTIFIED

Once you have determined potential risks to your patient protected health information, you must work toward solutions to decrease those risks, addressing the items that are of highest risk first. This is typically referred to as a risk mitigation or risk remediation plan.

Sanction Policy

✪ **Has your organization implemented a sanction policy to apply to your workforce who fails to comply with security policies and procedures? Has the workforce been trained on the policy?**

Sanction Policy (45 CFR §164.308(a)(1)(ii)(C)), (Required). A sanction policy must be in place to apply appropriate sanctions to the organization's workforce who fail to comply with your policies and procedures protecting security of your PHI. This can become part of your human resources policy. The workforce should be trained on policies and procedures and have clear guidance on how violations will be handled by administration. Sanctions may range from a verbal reprimand to termination, which adjust the disciplinary action based on the severity of the violation. A range of examples should be offered such as verbal or written reprimand, retraining on policies and procedures, suspension, or termination. Workforce members should be educated that there are both civil monetary penalties and criminal penalties, including incarceration provided under HIPAA or other applicable law. It is recommended that workforce members be required to sign a statement that they have received this training and agree to security policies and procedures. A social media policy is recommended.

Sanction policies and procedures can also be included in your security awareness training program. All sanctions should be documented with the outcome included.

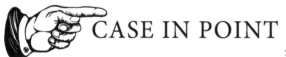

⊕IPAA
DEMYSTIFIED

You must have a sanction policy in place in your practice in the event a member of your workforce accidentally or intentionally violates your privacy and security policies and procedures. Be sure to give examples of violations that can occur via portable media devices (e.g., smart phones) as well as improper posting to social media.

CASE IN POINT
74

In 2007, 27 employees were suspended without pay for a month for violating HIPAA regulations. Employees at the Palisades Medical Center in North Bergen, New Jersey, violated HIPAA regulations by peeking at the medical records of George Clooney, who had been brought in with a companion after the pair had a motorcycle accident. Palisades operated according to its own sanction policy by suspending the workers who did not "need to know" Clooney's medical information.

Information System Activity Review

✪ **Does your organization implement procedures to regularly review records of information system activity such as audit logs, access reports, and security incident tracking reports?**

Information System Activity Review (45 CFR §164.308(a)(1)(ii)(D)), (Required). Policies and procedures for an information system activity review must be made with procedures to regularly review records of your information system activity, such as audit logs, access reports, and security incident tracking reports. Information system activity needs to be regularly reviewed, and you will want to be able to understand the audit and activity review functions and computer systems, monitor system activity (e.g., log-in attempts, discrepancies), and generate logs of system activity, all of which are done on a regular basis and documented. Logs of any security incidents should be kept for six years.

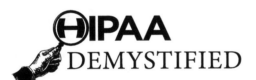

⊕IPAA
DEMYSTIFIED

Your IT person or department must have a way to monitor for and track potential breaches of electronic protected health information (EPHI). If you have consistent monitoring, it is much easier to understand when there are irregularities that may cause a breach of EPHI. For example, these logs may be helpful in identifying hacking attempts or other improper access to your systems housing EPHI.

Assigned Security Responsibility

✪ **Do you have a chief security officer for your practice or organization? Does your workforce know the name and contact information of this person or department?**

Assigned Security Responsibility (45 CFR §164.308(a)(2)), (Required). You must assign security responsibility and name a chief security official who is responsible for security and implementation of the security policies and procedures. While you need one individual who is designated as your chief security official who has overall responsibility for security regulations, you may assign other individuals for specific tasks or responsibilities. For example, you may have someone who manages security of the building, while another manages your network security. Be sure all staff knows who these people are and how to contact them.

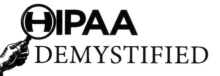

You must assign a chief security official to monitor compliance with the security regulations and to be available to respond to any breach. This person may be the same person as the chief privacy officer, but need not be.

Workforce Security

✪ **Does your organization have policies around who can access EPHI and under what conditions, as well as policies and procedures to prevent workforce members from obtaining access to EPHI that is not within their duties? Does your organization define roles and responsibilities to assure that no one person has too much authority?**

Workforce Security (45 CFR §164.308(a)(3)), (Required Standard). CEs need to implement policies and procedures that ensure the workforce has appropriate access to EPHI, with the minimum necessary access required for the workforce member to do his or her job. Workforce needs access to EPHI to carry out their duties; policies and procedures need to identify the EPHI that is needed, when it is needed, and control access to EPHI. A CE must control access to EPHI such that it knows what EPHI is needed and when it is needed. A CE should be able to list all of its BAs and the access that each requires to its facilities, information systems, electronic devices, and EPHI.

HIPAA DEMYSTIFIED

You must determine which person or job role can access electronic protected health information (EPHI), what EPHI they may access, and when it is needed (i.e., the roles and privileges of each workforce member). Business associates are also subject to this requirement.

Authorization and/or Supervision

✪ **Does your organization have policies and procedures in place to determine if workforce members' access to EPHI is appropriate for their job functions? Are there policies and procedures with regard to facilities, information systems, electronic devices, and EPHI?**

Authorization and/or Supervision (45 CFR §164.308(a)(3)(ii)(A)), (Addressable). You must implement procedures for the authorization and/or supervision of workforce members who work with EPHI or in locations where it might be accessed; policies and procedures must be implemented to ensure all of your workforce has appropriate access to EPHI as needed, while preventing access those workforce members who do not need to access EPHI, or particular types of EPHI. Only those workforce members who have a "need to know" should have access to EPHI; role-based access is recommended. Roles and responsibilities for all job functions must be assigned, and duties must be identified for each workforce member or job function, identifying what EPHI is needed, and when it is needed. You also need to have procedures for authorizing system users and changing authorization permissions. You need to have clear chains of command with staff aware of the identity and roles of their supervisors. In small practices or offices, all workforce members may need access to EPHI to do their jobs.

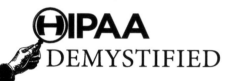

You need to decide what staff in your practice should have access to protected health information and determine access that gives them the minimum necessary to do their job. Business associates are also subject to this requirement. This allows the covered entity to meet the minimum necessary requirement discussed in chapter 4. Minimum necessary does not apply when disclosures are needed for treatment purposes, when releasing information to the patient or their representative, or when a patient authorizes release of their health information.

Workforce Clearance Procedures

✪ Have all of your workforce members received appropriate clearances prior to accessing patient information? For example, have their background and credentials been verified? Do you have procedures for granting or terminating access to EPHI?

Workforce Clearance Procedures (45 CFR §164.308(a)(3)(ii)(B)), (Addressable). Organizations need to address whether all members of the workforce with authorized access to EPHI receive appropriate clearances. CEs must establish procedures to verify that a workforce member has clearance to access EPHI for their job function. Policies and procedures should require appropriate screening of workforce members prior to accessing facilities, information systems, and EPHI. HIPAA compliance training for workforce should be made available prior to access to EPHI.

ⒽIPAA
DEMYSTIFIED

The identity and credibility of your workforce must be established prior to having access to confidential information paper protected health information and electronic protected health information. This may include background checks or other workforce screening measures.

Termination Procedures

✪ **If a workforce member quits or is terminated from a position, are there policies and procedures in place to terminate access to your facilities, information systems, and EPHI? For example, have access privileges to your data resources been revoked? Has all hardware, software, and data been retrieved from the workforce member? Does your organization have policies and procedures in place for when a BA is terminated?**

Termination Procedures (45 CFR §164.308(a)(3)(ii)(C)), (Addressable). CEs need to implement procedures for terminating access to EPHI when the employment of a workforce member ends. Procedures may differ for voluntary terminations versus involuntary terminations.

Procedures should be established regarding recovery of keys, identification badges, access cards, and so on, as well as deactivating computer access, such as user IDs and passwords. Clearance changes must also be considered for limiting access in situations such as demotion, which may bring a change in access rights.

⊕IPAA
DEMYSTIFIED

When workforce members leave your practice, be sure their access to any Electronic Protected Health Information (EPHI) is terminated and any EPHI data sources are returned. Business Associates are also subject to this requirement. Be sure any portable media devices have been returned and/or wiped.

Information Access Management

✪ **Does your practice have policies and procedures that describe how to limit access to EPHI?**

Information Access Management (45 CFR §164.308(a)(4)(i)), (Required Standard). You must implement policies and procedures for authorizing access to EPHI, based on the workforce member's role. Computer systems and applications that provide access to EPHI must be identified, with access controlled based on job role or function.

HIPAA
DEMYSTIFIED

You must restrict access to Electronic Protected Health Information (EPHI) in your computer system by job responsibilities, allowing access only to persons or software programs that must have the named EPHI to do their job.

Clearinghouse Functions

✪ **If you have a Health Care Clearinghouse (HCC) in your organization, is access to EPHI separated from the rest of your organization?**

Clearinghouse Functions (45 CFR §164.308(a)(4)(ii)(A)), (Required). An HCC is an entity that processes raw data it receives into an electronic health transaction, or vice versa, depending upon what is needed. If an HCC is part of a larger organization, the HCC must implement policies and procedures that protect the EPHI of the clearinghouse from unauthorized access by the larger organization. In the unlikely event an HCC exists within your organization, you must implement procedures for accessing EPHI that are consistent with the HIPAA Privacy Rule. That is, you must prevent access by the clearinghouse the same way you would prevent access by any other outside entity. If you do not house or depend upon a clearinghouse, document this fact to satisfy your HIPAA requirement.

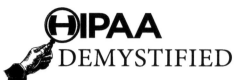

Health Care Clearinghouses (HCCs) are entities that process nonstandard health information they receive from another entity into a standard (i.e., standard electronic format or data content), or vice versa. You are very likely not a HCC and are not subject to this regulation. Document this fact.

Access Authorization

✪ **Does your organization have policies and procedures that explain how it grants access of EPHI to its workforce and to other entities such as BAs (possibly based on job function)? Is it documented? Do you have authorization and clearance procedures in place?**

Access Authorization (45 CFR §164.308(a)(4)(ii)(B)), (Addressable). You must implement policies and procedures for granting access to EPHI. You need to determine what person or system should be authorized to have access to EPHI, when you grant access privilege, and the process by which they can access EPHI.

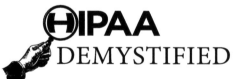

You need to know WHO can access protected health information, WHEN they can do it, and HOW you are going to facilitate it and keep track of it. This information needs to be documented in your organization's policies and procedures. Workforce need to be trained on appropriate access to protected health information.

Access Establishment and Modification

✪ **Does your organization have policies and procedures that address who, when, where, and how an individual or other entities (e.g., BAs) gain access to EPHI? Does your organization have policies and procedures that establish, review, and modify a user's access to EPHI? Is it documented? If your workforce can access EPHI from alternate locations, what method of access controls is used?**

Access Establishment and Modification (45 CFR §164.308(a)(4)(ii)(C)), (Addressable). A CE must have policies and procedures that establish, review, and modify a workforce member's right to access a workstation, transaction, program, or process; all must be documented and periodically reviewed and updated as needed. Policies and procedures should explain how your organization assigns privileges to EPHI; there is typically segregation of duties. Generally, access is granted to the point that a workforce member has access to the minimum necessary EPHI to do their job. User rights should be reviewed, documented, and modified if the user's rights change. In a therapy practice, access authorization might include measures such as limiting user's access to their assigned caseload. Access rights can be granted based on the workforce's identity, roles, location, or a combination therein. Workforce should be trained on HIPAA security awareness prior to obtaining access to EPHI.

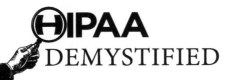

Your practice needs policies and procedures determining who can access particular electronic protected health information (EPHI), how they can access it, and from where they may access it. Workforce must only have access to EPHI which is necessary to do their jobs. Remote access policies and procedures should be developed if people access EPHI remotely.

Security Awareness Training

✪ **Does your organization offer security awareness training to new and existing members of the workforce? Is there periodic retraining of the workforce, including management, when there are changes that affect the security of EPHI?**

Security Awareness and Training (45 CFR §164.308(a) (5)), (Required Standard). Your organization needs a training program that makes each individual with access to EPHI aware of the measures you have in place to reduce the risk of improper access, use, and disclosure of EPHI. Training should also include specific role-based training. In addition, periodic retraining should occur when environmental or operational changes occur that affect the security of EPHI. This may be new security technology, upgraded software or hardware, or changes in the Security Rule. Records of all training materials, sign-in sheets, quiz results, and so on should be retained for six years.

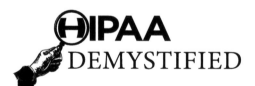

The workforce in your practice, including management, need to be trained on security policies and procedures related to their job, with retraining when there are material changes to your operations or the regulations. Training materials should be kept for six years; all materials should be dated to facilitate this process.

Security Reminders

✪ **Do you give regular, timely security reminders and updates to your workforce? These reminders can take the form of a meeting, email reminders, bulletin board postings, and so on.**

Security Reminders (45 CFR §164.308(a)(5)(ii)(A)), (Addressable). Security reminders can take many forms—agenda items for meetings, email reminders, bulletin board postings, and so on. Information can include reminders and updates on virus protection, malicious software, as well as password protection.

⊕IPAA
DEMYSTIFIED

You must determine how to educate your workforce regarding electronic security precautions. This may include reminders to not share user IDs, or directions for creating strong passwords. Other areas of reminders may concern issues such as encryption, transmitting electronic protected health information, screen savers, and instructions on logging off and locking computer systems. Keep documentation regarding these reminders for six years.

Protection from Malicious Software

✪ **Does your organization have anti-malicious software installed and regularly updated? Is there a way to scan attachments and downloads for malicious software? Is the workforce trained on guarding against, detecting, and reporting malicious software?**

Protection from Malicious Software (45 CFR §164.308(a)(5)(ii) (B)), (Addressable). Unauthorized infiltration can cause EPHI to be damaged or destroyed. CEs must implement procedures for guarding against, detecting, and reporting malicious software (e.g., viruses, Trojan horses, and worms). Software patches and antivirus software should be implemented. Default logins and passwords should be removed from the IT system, unnecessary services disabled, and ownership permissions set. Perform network vulnerability scans on systems containing or accessing EPHI, install firewalls, and consider intrusion detection software if reasonable and appropriate. Workforce members need training on types of threat (e.g., phishing, malware) and what to do about them.

⊕IPAA
DEMYSTIFIED

Workforce must be trained to protect their computer and other electronic data devices from viruses and malware and to regularly backup files. This includes information on how to avoid falling victim of phishing attacks, virus protection, and what to do should malicious events occur.

Log-in Monitoring

✪ **Do you have a procedure for monitoring log-in attempts, as well as detecting and reporting discrepancies? Is it part of your security awareness training program?**

Log-in Monitoring (45 CFR §164.308(a)(5)(ii)(C)), (Addressable). You must institute a procedure for monitoring log-in attempts and detecting and reporting discrepancies. An inappropriate or attempted log-in occurs when someone enters multiple combinations of usernames and/ or passwords to gain access to an information system. Most information systems allow for a set amount of unsuccessful log-ins before it locks a user out. If it is reasonable and appropriate, documentation of these attempts may be logged. Overall, the purpose is to make workforce members aware that multiple log-in attempts are not appropriate.

ⒽIPAA
DEMYSTIFIED

Workforce should be trained on log-in procedures and the danger of sharing passwords. IT should monitor access to the electronic protected health information system, and enable a process that eliminates access when risks such as multiple attempts to login with an incorrect password occur.

Password Management

✪ **Do passwords get changed on a regular interval? Do you train your workforce on creating strong passwords and safeguarding passwords? Is it part of your security awareness training program?**

Password Management (45 CFR §164.308(a)(5)(ii)(D)), (Addressable). Policies and procedures are needed for creating, changing, and safeguarding workforce passwords. The NIST notes that evaluation for password strength includes the password's complexity and length and having users know how to create and safeguard a secure password. Policies and procedures should be in place to prohibit password sharing, as well as instructions regarding writing down and storing passwords. Password managing should be part of your security awareness training.

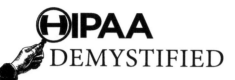

HIPAA DEMYSTIFIED

Train your workforce on strong passwords that cannot be easily guessed or cracked, and prohibit password sharing and writing down of passwords. IT should establish a schedule by which passwords must be changed.

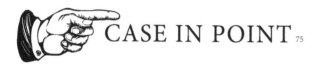

CASE IN POINT 75

After reality TV star Kim Kardashian gave birth in 2013 at Cedars-Sinai Medical Center, six workers were fired for inappropriate access to the hospital's electronic health records system. Four physicians shared access privileges, logins, and passwords with their employees; five employees subsequently used the user names and passwords of the physicians to inappropriately peek at medical records for patients who they had no role in treating. The physicians were fired and barred access from the Cedars-Sinai electronic health record system, even if they work for another provider in the future. A medical student and an unpaid student medical research assistant were also fired.

Security Incident Response and Reporting

✪ Do you have policies and procedures for addressing security incidents? Do they list possible types of security incidents, how they should be handled, and to whom they should be reported?

Security Incident Response and Reporting (45 CFR §164.308(a)(6)(ii)), (Required). You must have a way to identify and respond to security incidents, mitigate any harmful effects from the incident, and document both the incident and the outcome. The incidents should align with your emergency response plan, with system recovery prioritized. Security incidents can range from virus attacks, to break-ins with theft of EPHI, unauthorized user access, and so on. CEs must develop procedures that assign roles and responsibilities for incident response so the appropriate workforce knows the course of action, which may include mitigating damage, documenting the incident, evaluating how the security incident occurred as part of the incident, as well as for ongoing risk management practices. Training should address prevention, detection, and incident response.

HIPAA DEMYSTIFIED

Have documented policies and procedures addressing security incidents and how to handle breach of protected health information (paper or electronic). Train your workforce on these policies and procedures; breach notification procedures should be followed if necessary.

Contingency Plan

✪ During an emergency, does your practice know what crucial services and EPHI must be available? During a natural or man-made disaster, does your organization have policies and procedures that cover damage to its information systems and potential threats posed to EPHI during an emergency?

Contingency Plan (45 CFR §164.308(a)(7)(i)), (Required). Policies and procedures required for responding to an emergency (e.g., fire, vandalism, system failure or a natural or man-made disaster) that damages systems containing EPHI, and updated and implemented as needed.

⊖IPAA
DEMYSTIFIED

Your practice should have an emergency response plan such that electronic protected health information is available to your workforce as needed, which takes into account IT problems, and potential natural disasters or disasters of human origin.

Data Backup Plan

✪ **Do you have a plan to back up your EPHI such that you can maintain and retrieve an exact copy of the EPHI? Have you considered all of your important sources of data (e.g., case records, accounting records, diagnostic information)?**

Data Backup Plan (45 CFR §164.308(a)(7)(ii)(A)), (Required). You must establish and implement procedures to create and maintain retrievable exact copies of EPHI in the event of an emergency or disaster (e.g., fire, flood, vandalism, system failure, natural disaster). Various methods of backup should be considered (e.g., tape, disk, CD, cloud storage), and backup copies should be stored in a physically separate location from the data source. Frequency of backups should be determined based on the needs of the CE. CEs should document the creation of backups and their storage.

⊖IPAA
DEMYSTIFIED

Keep frequently updated backup copies of your practice's electronic protected health information (EPHI). If your EPHI is not cloud based, keep backups in a separate location from the primary workplace.

Emergency Mode Operation Plan and Disaster Recovery Plan

✪ **If there is an emergency, can you access your EPHI? In the event electronic access is unavailable, are there manual procedures for security protection that can be implemented if needed? Do you have a way to protect and reinstate EPHI in the event of an environmental catastrophe (e.g., fire), a natural disaster (e.g., flood or earthquake), system failure, or criminal activity?**

Emergency Mode Operation Plan (45 CFR §164.308(a)(7)(ii) (C)), (Required) and **Disaster Recovery Plan** (45 CFR §164.308(a)(7) (ii)(B)), (Required). You are required to establish procedures to enable continuation of critical business processes for protection of the security of EPHI should you have a crisis or emergency. Procedures should enable continuation of critical business processes for protection of the security of EPHI while operating in emergency mode, while simultaneously keeping EPHI secured. You must establish and implement procedures to create and maintain retrievable exact copies of EPHI. Specific issues of the plan include what data is to be restored and how it is to be restored. A copy of the plan should be readily available and ideally at more than one location. Data protections (firewalls, patches, etc.) should be reapplied before complete restoration of EPHI.

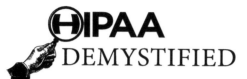

Have security protections in place in the event of power or technical failure, evacuation, or other crisis or emergency. Designated roles and responsibilities should be clear, and contact information should be available to the workforce.

Testing and Revision Procedures

✪ **Have you tested out (and revised as necessary) your data backup plan, emergency operations plan, and disaster recovery plan? Have necessary corrections been made? Has it been documented?**

Testing and Revision Procedures (45 CFR §164.308(a)(7)(ii)(D)), (Addressable). You must implement procedures for the periodic testing and revision of contingency plans, based on what is reasonable and appropriate for the size of your organization and costs to implement the procedures. CEs should test their contingency plan regularly, revise it as necessary, and make sure the workforce is aware of the plan. Each involved workforce member should understand the responsibilities.

⊖IPAA DEMYSTIFIED

Periodic training and testing of contingency plans should occur; revisions should be made based on feedback after testing the plan. Workforce members should understand their role in the plan. Trial runs are encouraged, with policies and procedures changing in response to the trial run process as needed.

Applications and Data Criticality Analysis

✪ Do you know what EPHI you would need the most in the event of an emergency? Have you identified your software applications and determined how important each is to patient care and daily business?

Applications and Data Criticality Analysis (45 CFR §164.308(a)(7)(ii)(E)), (Addressable). You need to implement an accounting of your technology resources for normal operations, as well as those needed during contingency operation. This includes your software, network data, or workstations: essentially any data applications that store, maintain, or transmit EPHI. Provisions must always be made for restoring these applications should there be an emergency. It is recommended that you develop a prioritized list for which software and data need to be available at all times and which would be restored first in the event of a contingency.

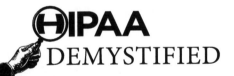

Practices need to prioritize what electronic protected health information (EPHI) and software applications have the highest priority for restoration after a crisis or emergency, with sequential policies and procedures for workforce to follow to gain access to the most critical EPHI for your practice.

Evaluation

✪ Do you perform both technical and nontechnical evaluations in response to environmental or operational changes in your organization that may affect the security of EPHI? When are evaluations done? Are they documented?

Evaluation (45 CFR §164.308(a)(8)), (Required Standard). Periodic evaluation reports of a person or role should be designated to be responsible for assessing risk and engaging in ongoing evaluation, monitoring, and reporting of security events. Internal or external reviewers should evaluate your organization. The effectiveness of security safeguards in your organization's physical environment, business operations, and information systems should be evaluated. For some larger CEs, it is reasonable and appropriate to conduct penetration testing to evaluate the security of your IT. This allows you to proactively manage existing vulnerabilities in your system to decrease the risk of breaches of EPHI. Once evaluation has occurred, results should be analyzed, security weaknesses corrected, and evaluations should be repeated periodically. Document your results.

(H)IPAA
DEMYSTIFIED

You must regularly assess risks to the security of electronic protected health information in your practice, with corrections made as needed, and your process documented. This process is the same for your paper protected health information.

Business Associate Contracts and Other Arrangements

✪ Do you have a BA contract or other written arrangement in place with your BAs? Does your organization identify a person or department responsible for making sure business associate agreements (BAAs) are in place prior to their access to EPHI? Do your BAs have contracts in place with their subcontractors?

Business Associate Contracts and Other Arrangements (45 CFR §164.308(b)(1)), (Required Standard); (45 CFR §164.314(a)(2)(i), 164.308(b)

(1)), (Required); (5 CFR 4 §164.314(a)(2)(i)), (Required). A CE may allow a BA to create, receive, maintain, transmit or store EPHI for the CE with satisfactory assurances that the BA will appropriately safeguard the information. Assurances can be done, in part, through the business associate agreement (BAA). The BAA or other written contract will state that the BA will implement appropriate administrative, physical, and technical safeguards that protect the PHI that it creates on behalf of the CE.

———————

A business associate (BA) is a person or entity that creates, receives, maintains, transmits, or stores protected health information (PHI) on behalf of a CE. Examples may be your attorney, billing service, accreditation, electronic health records vendor, IT company, and document shredding service. If the service creates, receives, maintains, transmits, or stores PHI on your behalf, they must also be compliant with the HIPAA regulations.

A subcontractor of a BA is an entity that creates, receives, maintains, transmits, or stores Electronic Protected Health Information (EPHI) on behalf of the BA and must also be compliant with HIPAA regulations. For example, if an electronic health records company, as a BA uses a cloud-based service from another company, the cloud-based service would be considered a subcontractor, who is then required to abide by the HIPAA privacy and security regulations.

———————

The BAA should also specify that any subcontractor of a BA also meets HIPAA requirements (CEs are not required to have a BAA or other written contract with a BA's subcontractors). BAAs are to specifically note that the BA or subcontractor are to report any security incident to the CE when it becomes aware of it, and the BAA is also written to authorize termination of the contract by the CE if the CE determines the BA has violated the terms of the contract. Contracts must describe the permitted and required uses of PHI by the BA. BAAs include stipulations that:

- describe the permitted and required uses of PHI
- the BA will not use or further disclose PHI other than as permitted or required by the contract or the law
- the BA will use appropriate safeguards to prevent use or disclosure of PHI
- the BA reports other uses or disclosures that occur outside of the agreement
- the BA gets assurances from any subcontractors to protect PHI
- when a CE knows of a breach or violation by the BA, the CE is required to take steps to cure the breach or end the violation, and if necessary, terminate the contract (or report the violation to HHS if termination is not feasible)
- PHI will be returned to BA upon termination of the contract.

If both the CE and the BA are both government entities, the CE can comply with the contract standard by entering into a Memorandum of Understanding (MOU) with the BA, or if other law requires the same privacy and security protections as HIPAA regulations. For government entities, the termination authorization may be omitted from the MOU if other law prohibits the termination.

If your organization is the BA of another CE, and you have subcontractors performing activities that involve EPHI, subcontractors should be required to provide satisfactory assurances of protection of

EPHI. Document the satisfactory assurances. It is recommended that a centralized list of BAs be kept with contract expiration/renewal dates. Sample BAAs are available at the HHS website, www.hhs.gov.

ⒽIPAA
DEMYSTIFIED

Business associate agreements or other written contracts must be in place documenting how electronic protected health information will be used and safeguarded. The agreements should be catalogued by expiration date, with a system established to monitor their status.

Summary

HHS defines administrative safeguards as "administrative actions, and policies and procedures, to manage the selection, development, implementation, and maintenance of security measures to protect EPHI and to manage the conduct of the covered entity's workforce in relation to the protection of that information."[76] The administrative safeguards are by far the largest of the three safeguards set by the security requirements and encompass administrative functions for management and execution of security measures.[77] All administration safeguards must be included in your SRA.

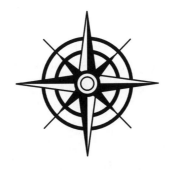

CHAPTER 10
Physical Safeguards

The physical safeguards of the security regulations are the physical measures, policies, and procedures to protect a covered entity's Electronic Protected Health Information (EPHI). These measures relate to protection of electronic information systems from natural and environmental hazards and unauthorized intrusion. They include facility access controls such as contingency operations, a facility security plan, access control and validation procedures, and maintenance records. It also includes workstation use and workstation security. Lastly, device and media controls are integral to physical safeguards including activities such as disposal, media re-use, accountability, and data backup and storage.

What follows are the physical safeguard requirements, with questions to guide your assessment of your security practices, and "demystify" this part of your security risk assessment. Each requirement must be included in your security risk assessment, with any needed changes documented in your risk mitigation plan (and appropriate action taken to correct the threat or vulnerability). If a requirement does not apply to your practice, you must document why it does not apply to you.[78,79]

Physical Safeguards

✪ **Does your organization have policies and procedures around implementing a security risk assessment (SRA). Have you considered risks to your IT system, including natural disasters, flooding, vandalism and burglaries?**

Physical Safeguards (45 CFR §164.316(a)), (Required Standard). Physical safeguards are policies and procedures devised to protect EPHI from physical threats such as unwanted access to your electronic database. Physical safeguards also ensure that you can access EPHI in emergencies. In protecting EPHI, it is prudent to implement reasonable physical safeguards for information systems and related equipment and facilities.

The Security Rule defines physical safeguards as "physical measures, policies, and procedures to protect an electronic information systems and related buildings and equipment, from natural and environmental hazards, and unauthorized intrusion."[78] All physical access to EPHI must be considered. This may extend outside of your office, including workforce members' homes or other locations where workforce access EPHI.

(H)IPAA DEMYSTIFIED

You must include all of your facilities and equipment that use, transmit, or store electronic protected health information electronic protected health information in your security risk assessment (SRA), this includes any mobile devices such as smart phones, tablets, laptops, and other types of digital assistance. Even if the devices are for personal use, if they contain protected health information, they need to be included in your SRA. Remember, as discussed in chapter 4, if there are any of the 18 identifiers that can be tied to a person, the information is considered protected health information.

Contingency Operations

✪ **In the event of an emergency (e.g., loss of power) or disaster (e.g., flood, tornado, or earthquake), do you have procedures in place to allow facility access while you restore lost data? Are appropriate workforce members allowed entrance to your facility so they can perform data restoration?**

Contingency Operations (45 CFR §164.310(a)(2)(i)), (Addressable). In the event of an emergency, you are required to establish and implement (as needed) procedures that allow facility access in support of restoration of lost data, under your disaster recovery plan and emergency mode operations plan. The goal is to maintain both security and access to EPHI while allowing for data restoration.

ⒽIPAA DEMYSTIFIED

It is wise to contemplate all potential eventualities should a crisis or emergency affect your practice, and plan accordingly. There should be virtually no way that your practice should not have data available in the event of a crisis, emergency, or disaster.

Facility Security Plan

✪ **Does your organization have safeguards in place to protect your facility (or facilities) from unauthorized access, tampering, and theft (e.g., locks, alarms, employee IDs)? Do you have written policies and procedures that detail what individuals have legitimate business needs to access your facility?**

Facility Security Plan (45 CFR §164.310(a)(2)(ii), (Addressable). Organizations need facility security plans, which are controls around who can have access to facilities and equipment that contain EPHI. For smaller organizations, this might be an area that is not routinely accessible to the public. Additional controls to consider that can prevent unauthorized access, tampering, and theft include locks on doors, alarms, surveillance cameras, and property control identifications such as engraving or tagging of equipment. For some facilities, it may also include a security guard. Visitor badges and escorts may be appropriate at some facilities.

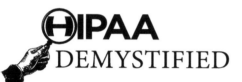

Document all of the security measures you have in place at your facility to deter unauthorized access to electronic protected health information, and update any methods or equipment needed. The more critical the data (e.g., psychotherapy notes), the more security measures should be in place. If your practice is in a high risk area, additional security measures may be warranted.

Access Control and Validation Procedures

✪ **Do you have policies and procedures in place that address who has access to your building (e.g., visitors and vendors), your software programs, and media containing EPHI with role-based access?**

Access Control and Validation Procedures (45 CFR §164.310(a)(2)(iii)), (Addressable). Your organization needs procedures to control who has particular access to buildings and areas that house systems or media containing EPHI. Access to information should be based on the role or function of the individual within the organization. Controlling access also means controlling visitor or vendor access. A vendor may need access to your software or computer system; a business associate agreement (BAA) should be in place if the entity has access to EPHI. For smaller CEs, workforce members may need access to all portions of the facility, including both paper and EPHI. In larger CEs, job functions will be more specialized and role-based access will need to be initiated. Access controls can include swipe cards, photo IDs, passwords or PINS, biometrics, or accompaniment by a security guard or control via a security camera. Sign-in sheets are also a form of access control and validation. For small organizations, access controls can be as simple as keeping visitors out of the reception and records areas.

(H)IPAA
DEMYSTIFIED

Establish or update policies and procedures that indicate WHO may have access to electronic protected health information (EPHI), WHEN they may have access, and from WHERE the EPHI can be accessed. For example, if your practice uses an electronic record system that can be accessed at home, you will want policies and procedures around who/when/how that data can be accessed outside of your office(s) so that privacy and security of EPHI is maintained.

Maintenance Records

✪ **Do you document repairs and modifications to the physical components of your facility?**

Maintenance Records (45 CFR §164.310(a)(2)(iv)), (Addressable). Policies and procedures should be developed detailing how you will document repairs and modifications to the physical components of the facility, which relate to security. This can include changing of locks, routine maintenance checks, and installing and maintaining security devices. Policies and procedures should specify all areas within your facility that require documentation. Documentation of maintenance should include the date the repair or modifications were made, as well as who made them.

(H)IPAA DEMYSTIFIED

Establish policies and procedures for who is allowed to do maintenance in your facility, how they get approved for access, and where they may go in your building(s). Maintain a log of who had access, what they did, and when they were in the building(s).

Workstation Use

✪ Do you have policies and procedures around access to workstations (e.g., desktop computers) in your facility? Do you have policies and procedures around mobile devices (e.g., laptops, tablets, and smart phones) and how and where EPHI may be transmitted, received, or stored on these devices?

Workstation Use (45 CFR §164.310(b)), (Required Standard). A workstation is defined as "an electronic computing device, for example, a laptop or desktop computer, or any other device that performs similar functions, and electronic media stored in its immediate environment" (45 CFR §164.304). This means your computer workstations but also any laptops, tablets, smart phones, and so on. If it can store or access EPHI, it is considered a workstation. You need policies and procedures that protect

PHI by safeguarding the physical surroundings of these devices that can transmit, receive, or store EPHI. Workstations that are fixed, such as a desktop computer, may be regulated by computer log-offs, as well as having screen protectors so those without access cannot see the screen. The organization should have policies about what types of EPHI can be accessed on portable devices (e.g., phones, tablets, laptops), rules about remote access (e.g., using secure channels), as well as what and how EPHI can be stored on these devices. Procedures should include the electronic devices, as well as the physical surroundings of the electronic devices.

⊖IPAA
DEMYSTIFIED

Establish inventory documentation of all electronic devices that store or can access to Electronic Protected Health Information (EPHI). Establish policies and procedures for both for monitoring the existence and location of the devices, as well as electronic procedures to ensure security of EPHI. Any maintenance of devices should also be recorded.

Workstation Security

✪ **Have you identified your wireless devices such as desktops, laptops, tablets, and any other portable or wireless devices? Do you have mechanisms in place for all devices that access EPHI so that access is restricted to authorized users? Is it documented?**

Workstation Security (45 CFR §164.310(c)), (Required Standard). This standard requires that CEs implement physical safeguards for EPHI to restrict access to authorized users. It includes desktop computers, as well as all wireless devices that access EPHI both at your facility and elsewhere. All workstation devices should be identified and logged (e.g., laptops, smart phones). Rules around unencrypted EPHI should be developed.

⊕IPAA DEMYSTIFIED

All potential access points to electronic protected health information (EPHI) should be documented, and policies and procedures should be developed. Establish inventory and documentation of all electronic devices that store or have access to EPHI. Establish policies and procedures for access to EPHI through these devices; encryption should be mandatory for devices that leave your facility.

Disposal

✪ Have you evaluated how you dispose of PHI/EPHI in your organization to render it unreadable or unusable? This includes paper records, computer CDs, USBs, tapes, smart phones, electronic memories in fax and copier machines, and other portable devices. Is your procedure documented?

Disposal (45 CFR §164.310(d)(2)(i)), (Required). Your organization must have policies and procedures in place that deal with the final disposition of PHI to render it unreadable, indecipherable, and unable to be reconstructed. Paper records need to be shredded, burned, or pulverized. For EPHI, policies and procedures clearing, purging, or destroying media is in order. Portable media must be included, which means any device capable of recording, storing, or transmitting data, voice, video, and photo images. Examples are laptops, smart phones, USBs, video cameras, pagers, and any other type of digital assistance mechanisms. Clearing means that it is overwritten with nonsensitive data, purging, or exposing the media to a strong magnetic field (also known as degaussing). Hard drive erasure software is also available. Destroying EPHI can include shredding, pulverizing, or incinerating the media (e.g., hard drive) on which EPHI is stored. Newer fax and copy machines typically store images it has transmitted on a hard drive; arrangements must be made for proper disposal of this EPHI as well. Media should be stored in a secure location prior to destruction. It is recommended that NIST standards be used.

(H)IPAA DEMYSTIFIED

Keep an inventory of all electronic devices that are used (practice owned and personally owned) that access electronic protected health information (EPHI). Develop policies and procedures about disposal of EPHI from these devices. Don't forget the electronic memory on your fax machine and copier!

Media Re-Use

✪ **Does your organization have policies and procedures in place for the removal of EPHI prior to reusing the media? Do you specify if the media can be re-used or if it must be destroyed?**

Media Re-Use (45 CFR §164.310(d)(2)(ii)), (Required). You must have policies and procedures addressing removal of EPHI from electronic media before the media is made available for re-use. You will want to consider whether use is for internal re-use (whereby re-imaging the media may be appropriate) or for external re-use, such as giving computers to a charity (whereby wiping the data may be appropriate).

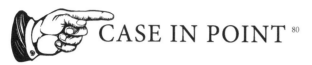

CASE IN POINT [80]

A New York not-for-profit managed care was informed by CBS news that they had purchased a photocopier previously leased by the organization. The breach included 344,579 individuals. The organization had returned multiple copiers to the leasing agents without erasing the hard drives. They were cited by the Office for Civil Rights not only on the breach of protected health information, but also for failing to implement policies and procedures that addressed returning of photocopiers.

HIPAA DEMYSTIFIED

Develop policies and procedures for media re-use that includes a specification as to whether devices that have been wiped may leave the facility or be re-used internally. Don't forget flash drives in your inventory of devices!

Accountability

✪ **Are you able to identify and track all of your media devices? Do you have a record of movements of and person(s) responsible for hardware or electronic media containing EPHI (e.g., hard drives, digital memory cards, magnetic tapes or disks, etc.)?**

Accountability (45 CFR §164.310(d)(2)(iii)), (Addressable). You must maintain a record of the movements of electronic media or hardware, documenting the person responsible for movement of media/equipment. If there are multiple devices of the same type, you must have a way to identify each device and log and record them separately (e.g., through serial numbers or another ID number). Policies and procedures about the transport of EPHI should be developed, and reporting of theft or loss of EPHI should be included. All types of hardware and electronic media must be tracked, including hard drives, magnetic tapes/disks, optical disks, digital memory cards, and so on.

HIPAA DEMYSTIFIED

All devices with electronic memory storage should be inventoried, detailing the item identification and the prescribed user of the device or storage mechanism. This inventory should be updated regularly as devices or workforce members change.

CASE IN POINT [81]

A billing company of a Medical and Mental Health Center in New York sent seven unencrypted CDs via a courier, which were subsequently lost. They were password protected, but unencrypted. Because they were not encrypted, and the loss involved over 500 records, a report had to be made to the Department of Health and Human Services about the loss of protected health information. Over 130,000 records were breached including social security numbers, addresses, dates of birth, health plan numbers, and driver's license numbers. Safeguards that would have prevented the breach include accountability (i.e. tracking of the data in transit), and encryption.

Data Backup and Storage

✪ **When you are ready to move equipment in your organization, do you have a way to create a retrievable, exact copy of the EPHI before you move the equipment? What is the process, and who is responsible for it? Is the process documented?**

Data Backup and Storage (45 CFR §164.310(d)(2)(iv)), (Addressable). Before moving equipment storing EPHI, you must be able to create a retrievable copy of EPHI when needed before movement of equipment. All data should be backed up in two or more physical locations.

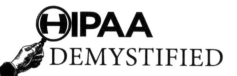

Back-up, back-up, back-up! Document where and how you backed up. Install software to automatically backup your electronic protected health information. You can use various backup tools such as online storage or system imaging. Do not store all data at one location. It is good practice to keep a backup copy to your backup copy. Document what information is important to backup, and what is not (e.g. program files or Windows folder).

Summary

Physical safeguards are policies and procedures developed to protect a CE's electronic information systems and related buildings and equipment from natural and environmental hazards and unauthorized intrusion. Standards under physical safeguards include facility access controls, workstation use, workstation security, and device and media controls.

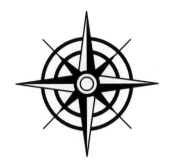

CHAPTER 11
Technical-Safeguards

Technical safeguards are the policies and procedures that practitioners use to protect Electronic Protected Health Information (EPHI) and control access to it. The Security Rule is based on fundamental concepts of flexibility, scalability, and technological neutrality; thus, no specific types of technologies are recommended by the U.S. Department of Health and Human Services (HHS). A covered entity (CE) must determine what is reasonable and appropriate for its own organization. Technical safeguards include access control measures, such as unique user identification, emergency access procedures, automatic logoff, and encryption and decryption. [82, 83]

What follows are the technical safeguard requirements, with questions to guide your assessment of your security practices, and "demystify" this part of your security risk assessment. Each requirement must be included in your security risk assessment, with any needed changes documented in your risk mitigation plan (and appropriate action taken to correct the threat or vulnerability). If a requirement does not apply to your practice, you must document why it does not apply to you.

—————•—————

A note about HIPAA compliance: HHS designed HIPAA to be "technologically neutral" as the government wished to facilitate the use of the latest and most secure technologies. There is no such thing as "HIPAA compliant" software, as you will often see advertised; HIPAA compliance is an ongoing process of maintaining privacy of Protected Health Information. Remember you may not ignore "addressable" specifications. Many of the addressable specifications were established when the technology to execute them was expensive. Today, it is much more affordable to comply with "addressable" specifications; practices have little excuse for not adopting them.

—————•—————

Access Control

✪ **Does your organization have policies and procedures for your electronic information systems, which govern the persons or software allowed to access EPHI?**

Access Control (45 CFR §164.312(a)(1)), (Required standard). You must have documented policies and procedures to specify which of your staff or which of your software programs should be granted access to EPHI.

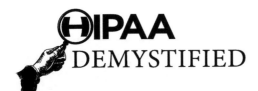

HIPAA DEMYSTIFIED

Determine who or what has access to what protected health information and how they have access, and establish policies and procedures to determine limiting access to the minimal necessary information to accomplish the intended purpose.

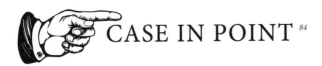

CASE IN POINT [84]

When Nadya Suleman (whom the media dubbed "Octomom") gave birth to octuplets in 2009, twenty-three employees at Kaiser Permanente Bellflower Hospital in Los Angeles improperly accessed her records. Fifteen employees were subsequently fired, and eight were disciplined. Transgressors ranged from orderlies to doctors. Kaiser Permanente was fined $250,000.

Unique User Identification

✪ **Does each user of your EPHI systems have a unique identifier to track their identity in your system?**

Unique User Identification (45 CFR §164.312(a)(2)(i)), (Required). Each user in your information system must have a unique identifier. This aids in holding users accountable for their actions by using a unique name and/or number to track that person in the system. There is no single format to establish user identification; CEs are free to develop any that suit their needs. Some CEs use a user name or a variation therein (e.g., jjones), but others use a set of random numbers and characters. The advantage to the latter is that it is less vulnerable to hacking efforts, but can be more cumbersome for the user.

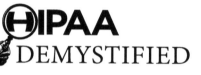

Determine policies and procedures for establishing user names or identification numbers, documenting the unique identifiers for your records. Unique user identifications is typically referred to as their "logon name" or "User ID." Nonactive workforce members User IDs should be removed or disabled.

Emergency Access Procedure

✪ **Do you have documented instructions and operational practices for obtaining access to EPHI during an emergency?**

Emergency Access Procedure (45 CFR §164.312(a)(2)(ii)), (Required). Define an emergency in your policies and procedures (for example, from a human threat or natural disaster). Establish procedures for obtaining necessary EPHI during an emergency, implementing as needed. Workforce members need instructions on when and how to access EPHI during these emergency situations. Emergency access procedures should not rely on any single person, nor should they rely on power or a network. There should be rapid access ability for workforce members who need information in the event of an emergency, and the ability for an audit log to be generated as a result of these situations.

⊖IPAA
DEMYSTIFIED

Imagine how you will operate during an emergency. The workforce should be able to "break the glass" as they would do for a fire alarm in the event of a fire, meaning staff should have rapid access to Electronic Protected Health Information (EPHI) in the event of an emergency. For instance, if there were to be a fire, flood, or vandalism, tornado, or system failure, how would workforce access EPHI?

Automatic Logoff

✪ Do your current information systems have an automatic log-off capability on all computers where EPHI is accessed?

Automatic Logoff (45 CFR §164.312(a)(2)(iii)), (Addressable). CEs need to implement electronic procedures to terminate an electronic session after a predetermined amount of activity. If a workstation is left unattended, automatic logoff decreases the possibility of inappropriate access to EPHI.

Encryption and Decryption

✪ The more sensitive the EPHI, the shorter the defined inactivity period should be before access is denied, requiring an individual to re-log into a system. For those with remote access, or for mobile devices, a time-out function should also be required. Do you use encryption methods to prevent access to EPHI by unauthorized people or software programs?

Encryption and Decryption (45 CFR §164.312(a)(2)(iv)), (Addressable). Encryption converts a text into encoded text (unreadable format) by use of an algorithm; decryptions decipher the encoded text into a readable format. Encryption creates a low probability that anyone other than the intended recipient will view the text. This implementation specification is addressable; you can decide based on what is reasonable and appropriate for your environment, taking into account the size of your organization, complexity, capabilities, technical infrastructure, cost, and risk. It generally makes sense to arrange to have your EPHI resting data encrypted, especially because price for encryption technology has significantly decreased. In addition, the majority of the most common security breaches involve portable data devices (e.g., laptops). While more costly, self-encrypting drives are an option, which is especially helpful for lost and stolen laptops.

Probably the most compelling reason to adopt encryption/decryption technology is the "safe harbor" provision set by the OCR, the entity that enforces the Health Insurance Portability and Accountability Act of 1996 (HIPAA) regulations. What this means is that if you lose EPHI or have it stolen and it is encrypted, it is not considered a breach and you are not required to report it to HHS. This fact alone makes investing in encryption technologies worthwhile. NIST provides guidance on encryption for data at rest, as well as data in transit.[85] Additionally, some states are now mandating encryption through state statute; for instance, Nevada now requires any "personal information of a customer" in transit be encrypted, with the exception of faxed data.[86]

Emails can also be encrypted, or communications between mail servers can be encrypted. Because encryption is an addressable specification, organizations can decide if adopting this technology is an acceptable cost. Lastly, some CEs opt for digital signatures on medical records, which are similar to encryption but cannot be unencrypted, providing authentication and nonrepudiation.

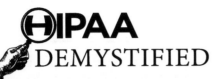

HIPAA DEMYSTIFIED

It is wise to encrypt your laptop and other portable electronic devices. Encryption gives you safe harbor if you have a breach, (meaning you do not need to report the loss or theft of data) and it is well worth the time and money invested. For small practices, encryption is now free in all versions of Windows 10 (and some versions of Windows 8), and easily accessed.

Audit Controls

✪ **Do you have hardware, software, or other procedural mechanisms that record and examine activity in your information systems that contain EPHI?**

Audit Controls (45 CFR §164.312(b)), (Required Standard). CEs must implement hardware, software, and/or procedural mechanisms that record and examine activity in information systems that use or contain EPHI; it does not specify what data must be gathered or how often audits should be reviewed. Your initial security risk assessment (SRA) should give you an idea of what types of controls or audit controls are needed to monitor EPHI. Most IT systems provide this capacity, and it is particularly useful if you believe EPHI has been wrongly accessed. Some CEs may find email-tracking systems useful, while others rely on email archiving.

Reviewing the audit process is part of risk management; this will include an examination of audit logs, which record sequential activities in an application or system or audit trails, which are logs where the system allows identification of a particular transaction or event. CEs will need policies and procedures as to what triggers an impromptu audit.

The date, time, patient identification, and user identification must be recorded when electronic health information is created, modified, accessed, or deleted, as well as an indication of which action(s) occurred. Triggers for internal audits may include a record of a patient with the same last name or address as the employee, VIP patient records (e.g., celebrities, political figures), high-profile events, patient files with no activity for 120 days, records with sensitive information such as psychiatric diagnoses, and so on.[87]

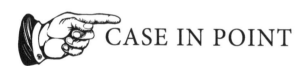

HIPAA DEMYSTIFIED

Your software vendor or IT person/department can run audit logs to check for unusual patterns of information that may be linked to breach or other potential problems. It is likely you already have this software in your system.

CASE IN POINT

A behavioral health organization was hit with Cryptolocker malware when an employee opened a phishing email. The malware encrypted the organization's data for which it had no key with which to decrypt the data. The organization was forced to pay a ransom of $1,000 on an anonymous site. Breached information included credit card information, birthdates, passwords, and driver's license numbers, which could still be sold lucratively on the black market even after the ransom was paid. The organization lacked basic audit controls such as audit logs and access reports, as well as data usage reports. The organization had not done the required security risk assessment, thus flaws in the required security risk assessment thus flaws in the covered entity IT system were unknown. The workforce was also not trained on security risks, so they lacked guidance on detecting and reporting malicious software. However, a sister organization was also hit with the Cryptolocker malware. Because it was able to review data usage reports, it was able to ascertain no data was breached and consequently was not required to report the event.

Integrity

✪ **Do you have policies and procedures in place to protect EPHI from improper alteration or destruction? Do your policies and procedures cover both technical and nontechnical sources of potential alteration or destruction?**

Integrity (45 CFR §164.312(b)), (Required). Workforce can make accidental or intentional changes that alter or destroy EPHI. Data can be altered or destroyed by human means or electronic media errors or failures. EPHI must be protected from being improperly altered or destroyed.

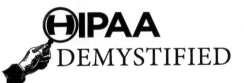

Make sure that you have clear policies and procedures for maintaining, altering, or destroying electronic protected health information. In many states, unauthorized alteration or tampering of medical records is illegal, with potential fines or jail time.

Mechanisms to Authenticate EPHI

✪ Does your organization have policies and procedures to protect EPHI from being accidentally or intentionally altered or destroyed from both technical and nontechnical (i.e., human) sources? Do you have a way to check whether your EPHI has undergone any unauthorized changes? Can your organization obtain a list of users denied authentication to your IT system?

Mechanisms to Authenticate EPHI (45 CFR §164.312(c)(2)), (Addressable). You must implement electronic mechanisms to substantiate that EPHI has not been altered or destroyed in an unauthorized manner. Integrity of data needs to be ensured; not doing so can put patient safety at risk. You will need a manner to detect, report, and respond to attempted or successful unauthorized modification or destruction of EPHI, which may include regularly reviewing access logs.

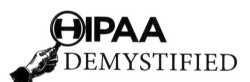

Authenticating electronic protected health information is both a technical and nontechnical process. The technical process can be accomplished with the use of continuous auditing; the nontechnical is training the workforce on policies and procedures to be proactive in inputting data correctly, as well as policies and procedures for when data must be corrected or amended.

Person or Entity Authentication

✪ Do you require a password, PIN, or other mechanism for the workforce to access EPHI?

Person or Entity Authentication (45 CFR §164.312(d)), (Required Standard). You must implement procedures to verify that a person or entity seeking access to EPHI is the person he or she claims prior to being allowed access to EPHI. Proof of identity is typically accomplished by a password or PIN, but can also be smart keys, tokens, or biometrics (e.g., fingerprints, voiceprints, facial patterns). Do not configure systems and applications to save passwords. The American Health Information Management Association notes there are categories of person or entity authentication:

- "Something you know – such as a password, or a shared secret (many systems now use one or more secret questions, the answer to which is only known by the user)

- Something you have – such as an identity token, a badge with an internal identification chip or bar code

- Something you are that makes you unique – such as a fingerprint, voiceprint, or retinal image."[88]

⊕IPAA
DEMYSTIFIED

For most practices, password protection suffices to protect data at rest. Workforce should be trained policies about creating strong passwords, not sharing passwords, or leaving documents or sticky notes in the workstation area with the password showing. Randomly generated passwords provide additional protection for sensitive data, but are typically used in industry, not health care practices.

Transmission Security

✪ **Have you encrypted your outgoing emails? Or have you stated in your policies and procedures that outgoing emails may not contain PHI?**

Transmission Security (45 CFR §164.312(e)(1)), (Addressable). As reasonable and appropriate, CEs must implement technical security measures to guard against unauthorized access to EPHI that is being transmitted over an electronic communications network. Patients do have the right to communicate by an alternative means. If a patient requests that you send EPHI by email, you can educate regarding the risks, but you are allowed to accommodate the client.

⊕IPAA
DEMYSTIFIED

Emails are governed by Access Control requiring you to have unique usernames and passwords), Person or Entity Authentication which requires you to ensure that only the intended recipients may access data, and Audit Controls which require you to produce audit trails of all sent and received emails). Emails must be secured during transmission, with each CE or BA determining if encryption of emails is reasonable and appropriate for their practice.

Integrity Controls

✪ **Does your organization have security measures to protect EPHI during transmission? Do you have some method to monitor that the data sent is the same as the data received (e.g., network communication protocols, data or message authentication codes)?**

Integrity Controls (45 CFR §164.312(e)(2)(i)), (Addressable). When reasonable and appropriate, a CE must implement security measures to ensure that EPHI is not improperly modified without detection while in transit. A CE's risk analysis should identify sources of threat to data integrity, and security measures should be implemented to protect data during transmission.

⊕IPAA
DEMYSTIFIED

Encryption is the best option for data in transit. However, small practices will want to consider whether encryption of emails is "reasonable and appropriate." Another alternative is to prohibit the transmission of electronic protected health information via email. Some providers opt for written permission from the client to email unsecured communication.

In Transit Encryption

✪ **Has your organization considered encrypting EPHI in transit?**

In Transit Encryption (45 CFR §164.312(e)(2)(ii)), (Addressable). The Security Rule allows CEs flexibility in determining when encryption is appropriate and with whom, as well as what method of encryption to use. The NIST provides guidance on encryption for data at rest, as well as data in transit at http://csrc.nist.gov.

⊕IPAA
DEMYSTIFIED

Your practice should evaluate whether encryption is a reasonable and appropriate standard for data in transit. There are commercially available platforms that encrypt email and text messages. When devices leave the office, it becomes data in transit, with a higher risk of breach. Encryption should be especially considered for laptops, portable digital devices, and USB drives, all of which have a heightened risk for loss or theft.

Summary

Technical safeguards protect and control access to EPHI. HIPAA regulations were designed to be technology neutral. No specific technology is required by the regulations; a CE may choose what best fits its practice. Technical safeguards include access control measures, unique user identification, automatic logoff, encryption, and decryption.

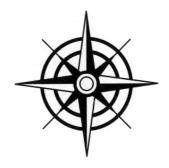

CHAPTER 12
Organizational, Policies and Procedures, and Documentation Requirements

Covered Entities (CEs) and Business Associates (BAs) have organizational requirements that include BA Agreements (BAAs), or some other contractual arrangement to protect electronic protected health information (EPHI). Additionally, each CE and BA must have documented policies and procedures, which may be kept in paper or electronic format. Documentation must be available to the workforce, and updated periodically.

Organizational Requirements[89]

Business Associate Contracts or Other Arrangements	• Business Associate Contracts (R) • Other Arrangements (R)

Table 12.1. Organizational requirements[90]

Business Associate Contracts or Other Arrangements

✪ Have you inventoried your Business Associate Agreements (BAAs) and do you know the expiration dates of your BAAs? Have you updated your BAAs with changes required by the Final Omnibus Rule of 2013?

Business Associate Contracts or Other Arrangements (45 CFR §164.314(a)(1), 45 CFR §164.314(b)(1)), (Required). Under the organizational requirements, you must account for your BAs, documenting that their contracts comply with the Security Rules. Business associate agreements (BAAs) or similar contracts should be updated to reflect changes of the Final Omnibus Rule of 2013. After the Final Omnibus Rule, BAs now include anyone who maintains/stores protected health information (PHI) in addition to the previous definition of "a person or entity that creates, receives, or transmits" PHI. Subcontractors of BAs must also comply with HIPAA regulations and make BAs liable for noncompliance by a subcontractor (making them eligible for civil and criminal penalties). "Other arrangements" refers to the ability to use a Memorandum Of Understanding (MOU) if the CE and BA are both governmental entities.

Policies and Procedures and Documentation Requirements

Policies and Procedures	• Required Standard 45 CFR § 164.316		
Documentation	• Time Limit (R) 45 CFR § 164.316(b)(2)(i) • Availability (R) 45 CFR § 164.316 (b)(2)(ii) • Updates (R) 45 CFR § 164.316 (b)(2)(iii)		

Table 12.2. Policies and procedures and documentation requirements

✪ **Do you have policies and procedures to comply with all of the standards, implementation specifications, and other requirements of the Security Rule?**

Policies and Procedures (45 CFR §164.316(b)(1)), (Required). Policies and procedures must be developed for each security standard, implementation specification, and other requirements. Policies and procedures can be changed at any time to meet the needs of your practice or modifications of the regulations, and also must be changed when there are material or operational changes in your practice.

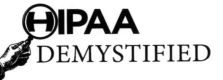

HIPAA DEMYSTIFIED

Policies are basic principles, rules, and laws your practice must follow; procedures define who does what, when, and under what criteria. You should address each standard and implementation specification in your policies and procedures by regulation number; in the event of an audit, you can more readily show you have addressed all of the regulations. Lastly, workforce members must be *trained* on relevant policies and procedures for them to be effective.

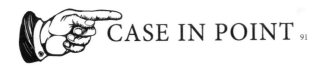

CASE IN POINT [91]

Personal data including names, social security numbers, and dates of birth for 26.5 million discharged veterans was stolen when a data analyst for the Department of Veteran's affairs improperly took the electronic data home. The analyst took home a laptop and an external hard drive, which were stolen from his home. Lawmakers told the VA that they need to fix "its broken data security system and failed leadership."

✪ **Do you have written or electronic documentation of your policies and procedures that you have implemented to comply with the regulations?**

Documentation (45 CFR §164.316(b)(1)), (Required). Documentation of the policies and procedures you use to meet the security regulations must be maintained. Documentation may include reports, assessments, investigations, sanctions, and training documents.

⊖IPAA
DEMYSTIFIED

As every practitioner knows, "if you didn't document, it didn't happen." This is also true for your HIPAA compliance program. In addition to making changes that enhance patient privacy and security, don't forget to document those changes in your policies and procedures.

Time Limit

✪ **Do you maintain your documentation for a minimum of six years?**

Time Limit (45 CFR §164.316(b)(2)(i)), (Required). A CE must retain required documentation for six years from the date of its creation or the date it was last in effect, whichever is later. This is a minimum retention period; documentation may be retained longer should state law, requirements of accreditation organizations, etc., require it. To aid in document retention, it is wise to include an effective date on your documents.

⊖IPAA
DEMYSTIFIED

Every documentation required by HIPAA regulations typically must be kept for a minimum of six years or longer, depending upon other requirements or needs in your practice. This does not include case records; HIPAA is silent on length of time medical or mental health records should be kept, deferring to any available state law.

✪ **Is documentation available to the pertinent workforce members?**

Availability (45 CFR §164.316(b)(2)(ii)), (Required). Documentation must be made available to workforce members who require it to do their jobs. The availability implementation specification requires CEs to "Make documentation available to those persons responsible for implementing the procedures to which the documentation pertains." Organizations often make documentation available in printed manuals and/or on Intranet.

⊕IPAA
DEMYSTIFIED

Keep documentation readily available to the workforce via printed manuals or an intranet website. Any updates must also be made available to the workforce.

Updates

✪ **Do you review your documentation periodically, updating it when there are operational or environmental changes to security of your EPHI?**

Updates (45 CFR §164.316(b)(2)(iii)), (Required). Documentation needs to be periodically reviewed and updated as needed.

⊕IPAA
DEMYSTIFIED

Periodic reviews and updates to your policies and procedures are needed because threats to electronic protected health information can change quickly; regulations, rules, policies and procedures also evolve.

Summary

Each CE must have BAAs or other written contract in place; MOUs can replace a BAA if both the CE and the BA are government entities. Every CE must have policies and procedures in written or electronic form, which must be readily available to the workforce who need it. Training of workforce on policies and procedures is essential to their success. Documentation must be kept for a (minimum) of six years, and periodically updated to meet environmental or operational changes.

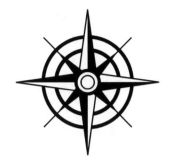

CHAPTER 13
Breach of Protected Health Information

The HIPAA regulations define *breach* as the "acquisition, access, use, or disclosure of PHI in a manner which compromises the security or privacy and protected health information."[92] Breach refers to unsecured PHI not rendered unreadable or indecipherable to unauthorized individuals. Data can be breached any number of ways; breach is most often promulgated by human error.[93] A lost or stolen computing device is the most common means of breach of PHI.[94] In 2014, theft of unencrypted storage devices and computer hardware used to store or access PHI accounted for the majority of data breaches; with laptop theft alone accounting for 25 percent of all incidents.[95]

In an analysis of HHS breaches of over 500 records, it was found that 38% of breach of PHI in 2015 was due to unauthorized disclosure (e.g. human error or improper access), 38% was due to theft or loss, 22% was due to hacking or an IT incident, and 2% was due to improper disposal. [96]

Breach due to unauthorized disclosure (38%) which can be attributed to human error or improper access, such as:

- In Indiana, a love triangle let Walgreens lost 1.4 million dollars in a judgment regarding inappropriate access of PHI. A pharmacist accessed pharmacy records of her boyfriend's ex-girlfriend to check for both birth control information and treatment for a sexually transmitted disease. [97]

- In Florida, 300 people being treated for depression were mailed free samples of Prozac. They had not given permission for this medical information to be released for marketing purposes. [98]

Examples of theft and loss (38%) include:

- Advocate Health Care group experienced the theft of four unencrypted laptops, breaching over 4 million records. [99]

- Horizon Healthcare Services, Inc., (Horizon Blue Cross BlueShield) experienced a laptop theft. While the laptops were physically secured, they were unencrypted. The loss was nearly 840,000 records. [100]

- Emmorton and Associates in Abingdon, Maryland, had a burglary with loss of paper PHI. Someone forced open a locked file cabinet in a counselor's office, which had paper PHI of 75 patients in it. Counseling records were potentially breached, including diagnosis and treatment information, social security numbers, dates of birth, home addresses and phone numbers, insurance information, and emergency contact information. [101]

Hacking or an IT incident (22%) accounted for 14 percent of breaches. For example:

- Choices, Inc., suffered a hacking incident that included one of their mental health facilities; 1,945 records were exposed. [102]

- The University of California Davis Health System was required to notify 1,326 patients when a physician's email was hacked. They were unsure how the email system was compromised. [103]

- A keystroke logger infected three computer's swiping the medical and financial data of 1,836 patients of the UC Irvine Student Health Center. The keylogger had been capturing and transmitting data to unauthorized servers for over a month before it was detected. [104]

Improper disposal (2%) include these examples:

- Just after the breach notification rule was instituted in 2009, it was discovered that CVS pharmacies were found to have disposed of patient PHI (records, pill bottles, etc.) in dumpsters. It occurred at so many sites that they were unable to estimate the loss of PHI. [105]

- The Carolina Center for Development and Rehabilitation suffered a breach when a doctor had his sons move his office. The sons mistakenly threw out 25 boxes of medical records, leaving them in a public recycling bin. There were 1,590 records involved. [106]

- A breach of 277,000 records occurred when a shredding company was hired by Texas Health Harris Methodist Hospital in Ft. Worth to shred decades-old microfiche medical records. Instead, the microfiche records ended up in a dumpster in a public park. [107]

Loss of the greatest *amount* of records is from hacking. The Anthem Breach of 2014 was the largest breach to date, with over 80,000,000 records being breached.[108] Breach of PHI is a significant problem, each CE must report actual breaches to HHS. Not all violations of privacy and security can be prevented; however, fines are typically predicated on how vigilant a CE was in their security efforts.

Exceptions to Breach

There are four instances where PHI may be disclosed in violation of the regulations but do not rise to the level of breach. They are incidental disclosures, unintentional access by someone internal to the CE, inadvertent disclosure to someone internal to the CE, and inadvertent disclosure to someone outside of the CE.

Incidental Disclosures. While practitioners can be careful not to disclose PHI, occasionally, in the course of business patients or others may hear "incidental disclosures" of PHI. Incidental disclosures are a byproduct of permissible or required disclosures and cannot reasonably be eliminated. They are not considered breaches as long as the provider has taken steps to minimize inappropriate use or disclosure of PHI through privacy safeguards, training of staff, and clear policies and procedures. For example, training staff to not discuss patients in the hallway would reduce incidental disclosures. Common incidental disclosures are sign-in sheets, names called in the waiting room, or a receptionist mentioning a name while scheduling an appointment.

Unintentional Access by Someone Internal to the CE or BA. In this situation a workforce member unintentionally acquires PHI in the scope of authority of their job, but the access does not result in further use or disclosures. For example, if a practitioner grabs the file of a patient of another staff member, but upon realizing their error, the practitioner hands the file back without reading the contents, it is not considered a breach.

Inadvertent Disclosure to Someone Internal to the CE of BA. For example, an internal email is sent to the wrong staff person, but the person who received the email alerts the sender and the email is returned or destroyed.

Inadvertent Disclosure to Someone External to the CE or BA.
A disclosure to someone outside of a CE or BA is considered a breach
except when it is reasonable to assume that the person would not have
been able to retain the information. For example, if you handed the results
of an assessment instrument to the wrong patient, quickly realize the
mistake, and retrieve the report.

Breach Notification Rule

The HIPAA Breach Notification Rule requires both HIPAA CEs and
BAs to provide notification following discovery of a breach of unsecured
PHI/EPHI. A breach is considered discovered on the day it is detected,
or when an entity reasonably should have known about the breach. CEs
and BAs must assume a breach unless they can demonstrate there is a low
probability that PHI/EPHI has been compromised. A risk assessment must
be conducted to determine if a breach has occurred.

Determining if a Breach Has Occurred

The Health Information Technology and Economic Clinical Health
(HITECH) Act requires a four-factor analysis of risk assessment for every data
security event, evaluating the probability that PHI has been compromised,
and the breach notification rule is triggered, or if the disclosure falls under
an exception to breach (see above). The following four factors are evaluated:

1. **The nature and extent of the PHI involved.** This includes the
   types of PHI identifiers and the likelihood of re-identification.
   The type of PHI is also considered: could the PHI be used in
   a manner that harms the patient? Does the breach fall under
   one of the exceptions to breach notification? (See exceptions
   to breach above.) Was the breach to another CE or BA? More
   sensitive information (e.g., psychotherapy notes, sexually
   transmitted disease information, substance abuse information)
   causes an increase in vigilance in evaluating the breach. Financial

information (e.g., social security numbers, birth dates, etc.) is also of increased concern.

If the EPHI that was breached was encrypted, unusable, or unreadable, the breach falls under the "safe harbor" exemption and does not need to be reported. Encryption methods must be in line with the National Institute of Standards and Technology (NIST) accepted methods.[109] With a Limited Data Set, (See Chapter 4) the probability of re-identification must be considered.

2. **The unauthorized person who used the PHI, to whom the disclosure was made, or who impermissibly accessed the PHI.** Does the person or entity have a legal obligation to protect the PHI? Has the information been accessed by someone who also is required to comply with HIPAA or other privacy laws? Has the information been breached by someone who could further exploit the PHI for their own interests?

3. **Whether the PHI was actually acquired or viewed.** Was there opportunity for the information to be acquired or viewed? Was the PHI recovered, and can it be proven it was not compromised in some way (e.g., acquired, viewed, transferred)?

4. **The extent to which the risk to the PHI has been mitigated.** A CE may take action to cure the breach, thereby lowering the probability of breach. For example, a CE may obtain satisfactory assurances that the information will not be used or disclosed further or will be returned or destroyed. This may be in the form of a written contract or confidentiality agreement.

When a potential bread occurs a risk analysis should be performed via the process described in chapter 8. The risk analysis can help you determine if you are facing low, medium or, high risk, or if the risk is not applicable to your operations. For breach analysis, *likelihood* refers to how likely the information could be impermissibly used or disclosed (high, medium, or low), and *impact* refers to how the loss of PHI could negatively affect the patient(s) (high, medium, low).[110]

A CE must demonstrate a low probability that the protected PHI has been compromised and document information relating to that conclusion. Based on your analysis, if you choose not to report the breach, documentation is important because you must establish the burden of proof. If there is a higher probability of breach, a breach response is necessary, prioritizing and mitigating identified risks.

Size of Breach and Necessary Response

If the breach involves fewer than 500 individual records or information, the risk assessment must be done to determine the level of potential harm and if you need to notify the individuals. CEs are required to assess the probability that PHI has been or may further be compromised based on a risk assessment. This assessment should look at (1) the nature and extent of PHI involved, (2) the person or entity who used the PHI or to whom the disclosure was made, (3) whether PHI was actually acquired or viewed, and (4) the extent to which the risk to PHI has already been mitigated.

When evaluating a potential breach, the practitioner should assess the cause of the incident, if indeed the incident meets the definition of a breach, conduct the risk assessment, and decide on what action to take (if any). As noted, the size of the breach affects how a CE must respond.

Breaches must be reported to patients without "unreasonable delay," and at least within 60 days of the discovery of the breach. Breaches of less than 500 records must be reported to HHS within 60 days of the end of the calendar year in which the breach was discovered. For a breach of over 500 individual records HHS must be notified within 60 days of the discovery of the breach. Local media must also be notified regarding the nature and extent of the breach, and you must post it on your website. Individuals are notified of breaches through first-class mail to the patient or the parent or legal guardian of the patient. If the patient is a minor, state law will dictate who has the authority to receive the notification.. If the individual is deceased, next of kin or a personal representative is notified. If individuals are unreachable, a substitute notice may be used. If the breach involves fewer than 10 individuals, a substitute notice may also be used in the form of a written notice, telephone call, or other means (e.g., website posting). For more than 10 individuals, you may post the notice on your website or other media, which includes a toll-free number (active for 90 days).

The content of the notice must include:

- a brief description of the breach and date of the breach and your discovery of the breach
- a description of what was breached
- steps the individuals should take to protect themselves
- a description of what you are doing in response to the breach and to prevent further breaches.

Contact procedures for more information needs to be included in the notice (e.g., toll-free telephone, email address, website, or postal address).

You must provide written notice by first-class mail or if the individual agrees by email (translation must be provided to those with English as a second language). If you do not have accurate contact information, you may provide a substitute notice. You must retain documentation regarding the investigation.

The Final Omnibus Rule clarifies that only contrary state laws are to be preempted by the federal breach law. That is, if it is impossible to abide by both state breach law and federal breach law, you are to follow federal breach law. You may also have additional responsibilities based on state law, the Fair Credit Reporting Act, or the Federal Trade Commission based on your organization's practices.

Business Associates and Breach

In addition, you are liable for breach of your contracted help, so BAAs are imperative. BAAs should specify the reporting of unauthorized uses and disclosures, incidents, and breaches to the CE, as well as the notification time period. Reporting to the CE must occur as soon as possible, but not more than sixty days from the date of discovery. If BAs do not comply with HIPAA regulations, termination of the contract should be considered or a report to the secretary of HHS may occur if termination is not feasible. Document any BA-related privacy or security issues.

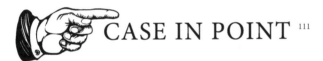 # CASE IN POINT [111]

> In a case of medical identity theft, Anndorie Sachs, a mother of four, received a call from Child Protective Services (CPS), who informed her she was under investigation because her newborn baby had tested positive for methamphetamines. Anndorie, however, had not given birth in years, nor had she ever used methamphetamines. CPS refused to believe her and started an investigation into her life, questioning her employers, her family, and her children. The thief, who had Anndorie's identification information, was a meth addict. She went to the hospital and gave birth under Sach's identity, starting the investigation into Anndorie's family life, as well as leaving her with a $10,000 hospital bill.

Costs of a Breach

As stated in chapter 1, fines for breaches can range from $100 to $1.5 million, and criminal penalties can include from one to 10 years in prison. The nature and the extent of the violation, the harm resulting from the violation, and a CEs history of compliance are all taken into consideration by the Office of Civil Rights when establishing penalties. Fines also vary depending upon when the violation occurred (changes occurred in 2009). However, penalties are not applicable if the CE was able to correct or cure the breach within 30 days after the person knew (or in exercising reasonable diligence should have known) of the violation.

Other potential costs may include reputational costs, for example from publicizing of the breach on the HHS website or via local media. Ethico-legal costs may arise from legal actions arising from state consumer protection laws, or civil lawsuits for violation of privacy. Lastly, the patient-therapist relationship may also be harmed when a CE is unable to maintain security of patient PHI.

Summary

Data breaches happen in numerous configurations, and every CE is likely to suffer a breach. In Ponemon's Privacy and Data Security study of 2012, 90 percent of survey participants had a data breach in the previous year.[112] Breaches happen in many manners, from unsecured laptops and electronic media devices (e.g., flash drives) to compromised IT, such as hacking, viruses, malware, improperly patched or outdated systems, and improperly configured or secured software. Improper disposal of PHI and device and media reuse can cause a breach. Mobile devices are of particular threat. Additionally, poor training may result in workforce inappropriately accessing PHI, which is considered a breach. Breach prevention is now considered the appropriate standard of care. Investing in data security improvements is a practical use of funds.

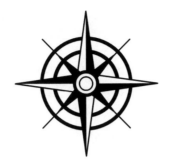

CHAPTER 14
Security Beyond Compliance

Threats to security of electronic protected health information (EPHI) evolve on a daily basis, in a way that could not have been envisioned in 1996, when HIPAA was enacted. Cybersecurity has since come front and center in our daily electronic lives. In this chapter, cybersecurity is introduced to give you an overview of security procedures to be aware of that go beyond just complying with the regulations. The goal of cybersecurity is to prevent, detect, or remediate an electronic security breach as quickly as possible. What follows is a discussion of various types of cyber attacks, as well as cyber defensive strategies for data at rest as well as data in transit.

Cyber Attacks

Malware. Malicious software damages or disrupts a computer system, potentially stealing information. It is commonly installed through email attachments, downloads of infected files, or infected websites. Downloading ActiveX technology can also introduce malware. Systems should be set to require confirmation that malware is absent in files and programs, before these files or programs are downloaded. Additionally downloaded files should be isolated from your network until you have assured yourself that malware is not present in these files.[113]

Protections include virus software, updated regularly, and scanning of attachments before downloading. Software security patches should be downloaded regularly; one option is to have a scheduled update day.[114] The workforce should be trained to recognize suspicious emails and avoid downloading files. Alternatively "white listing" applications can be used, which limits specific domains or programs that your system can accept. Policies and procedures should call for backup of files regularly.[115]

Phishing, Spear Phishing, and Whaling. Phishing is when a cyber-intruder seeks to access your personal information or passwords by posing as a business or organization with legitimate reason to request information, usually via an email or text that appears genuine. Spear phishing is an attack that targets a specific individual or business, while whaling is an attack aimed at a senior official in an organization.

The workforce should be trained to never provide their passwords to anyone via email, respond to requests for personal information, or open emails that contain spelling or grammar errors or are from an unexpected source.[115]

Hacking and Keyboard Logging. While hacking is not the most common cause of loss of Protected Health Information (PHI), it does result in the largest amount of loss of PHI. Hackers first gain access to a network, typically through a phishing email, whereby some or all of the found data is exported.[116] Keyboard logging involves software that tracks your actions on a keyboard, typically with intent to collect private data. Keyloggers get installed when you open a file attachment sent via email, text message, instant messaging, or social networks or by visiting an infected website.[117] Networks need to be well protected; prevention efforts may include a two-step authentication, a virtual keyboard, or a password generator.[118]

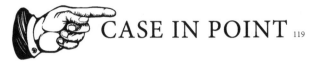

CASE IN POINT [119]

> Across the country, 4.5 million individuals from 206 hospitals, across 29 states had their personal information hacked by a group known as "Apt 18." They are suspected of stealing names, addresses, social security numbers, birthdays, and telephone numbers. One of the health systems stated that it believed that a foreign-based group out of China dispatched the malware looking for intellectual property.

Spam. Spam is advertisements that are distributed typically sent via emails, which may link you to phishing websites or install malware.[120] The workforce should be trained not to click on spam or download any attachments from spam mail. For some practices, an investment in spam filters may be a viable option.

Cookies. Cookies is a mechanism that allows a server to store its own information about a use on the user's computer, potentially tracking the activities of users over time and across different websites, putting personal information at risk. The workforce should be sure websites that ask for personal information are encrypted and the URL begins with "https."[121,122]

Denial of Service Attacks. Denial of service attacks are automated scripts that launch massive numbers of emails or calls to a website to such an extent that the victim is rendered useless. Prevention and solutions to denial of service attacks is more complicated than can be discussed here; the National Institute of Standards and Technology (NIST) offers a *Guide to Intrusion Detection and Prevention Systems (IDPS).*[123]

Crypto Wall. Crypto wall is software, typically introduced via a phishing attack that encrypts the victim's hard drive. Once encrypted, the victim is strong armed to pay a ransom to receive the encryption key so the victim can decrypt the hard drive and access the data. Additionally, in many cases, the crypto wall software simultaneously injects other malware to the system. A common situation is to inject keystroke logging malware which renders security systems ineffective.

Workforce members should be trained to not open emails that are suspicious, and covered entities (CEs) should have good backups for all devices connected to the network.

Guarding Against Lost or Stolen Data

In addition to the protections mentioned above, there are additional recommendations for data security, for data at rest, or for data in transit.

Encryption

Encryption is defined as the use of an algorithmic process to transform data into a form in which there is a low probability of assigning meaning without use of a confidential process or key.[124] It transfers plaintext (i.e., your document) into ciphertext, whereby you need a key to transfer the ciphertext back into data (i.e., decryption).[125] NIST outlines processes available for encryption for data at rest, and encryption for data in motion.[126] Encryption is not required under the regulation; however, if after a risk assessment, a CE determines that it is a reasonable and appropriate safeguard, it should be implemented. If not, the CEs should document what measures have been implemented instead.[127]

Encryption software may be purchased, but encryption is available through smart phones, note books, laptops and other computers. Risk assessment can help determine the level of encryption protection a practice needs. Because portable devices are one of the largest amounts of data breaches, encryption is highly recommended. It is suggested you encrypt patient data on your server, and avoid keeping patient data on stationary PCs.[128]

Encryption of Mobile Devices

In a Ponemon Institute study, 88 percent of the organizations allow their workforces to use their own mobile devices, yet 49 percent of the providers surveyed had not implemented security measures for the devices.[129] Most organizations in the Ponemon study of 2013 indicated they did not mandate encryption or antivirus or anti-malware software on the devices. Given that mobile devices are the most common source of breach, they should be encrypted.

Additional Cyber Defensive Strategies

In their book, *Successfully Choosing Your EMR: 15 Crucial Decisions*,[130] Arthur and Betty Gasch give excellent cyber-defensive advice. In addition to the techniques listed above, the Gasches advise the following:

Configure Computers Properly. Users should enable standard file sharing, disable guest user accounts on the system, and disable user-level registry access. Additionally users should lock down Windows installer except to administrators, activate system file protection, deploy a bidirectional firewall, and configure browsers for high security.

Limit Internet Access. It is recommended internet access be discontinued after office hours. Additionally, CEs should forbid internet surfing, games, and downloaded screen savers.

Incorporate Surveillance. Users should monitor access logs, and in larger organizations, consider penetration testing.

Cyber Insurance. Cyber insurance can offset costs of a breach and provide tools in the event of a breach notification. Policies should be read carefully. Business associates are typically not included, yet CEs are responsible for data breaches caused by business associates. Additionally, there may be exclusions if entities were not following HIPAA regulations.

Password Protection. Passwords should be at least eight characters in length and should contain a capital letter, a lowercase letter, a number, and a special character (%$*?!). For those with difficulty remembering, you can make a phrase or song to create a unique password, such as "Back2Square1!" , "$2donuts", or "Dontworry,Bhappy!"[131] Additional protection may include password encryption and vault storage.

Two-Factor Authentication. Two-factor authentication requires a second layer of log in. Typically when the first level log-in occurs (user name and password) a temporary second authentication key is delivered to the user, i.e., a text message will be sent to the user's cell phone. This authentication key has a short life (must be used within 20 minutes) for it to remain valid. Typically, these systems can be configured such that the second factor is required after a set number of days or when a logon is attempted from a new device.

Training of Workforce on Cyber Security. One of the biggest risks to e-security is lack of training for the workforce on computer/internet policies and procedures. CEs will want to train workforce on cyber-security, sending or posting regular reminders and updates.

Social Media

Social media is an excellent tool for education, advertising, and consultation with other professionals. However, it can also be a source of damaging privacy violations. There are many sources of social media to consider (e.g., Facebook, Twitter, LinkedIn, Tumblr, Google Plus, Instagram, Pinterest).[132] Insurion gives the following advice for using social media:[133]

- Assume that all of your social media activity is public

- Don't post about your clients, positively or negatively

- Be professional; inappropriate personal pictures can damage your image as well as that of your profession

- Keep professional and personal social media accounts separate

- Don't add clients to your social media accounts

- Don't use location check-ins if you are out in the field visiting patients.

Practices should have clear social media policies, with clear and consistent training on them.

Text Messaging and Emailing

Text Messaging. Many providers use text messaging to confirm or change appointments, or for quick check-ins with clients, among other uses. Texting has definite clinical advantages, but also brings security concerns. Texts may remain in a phone for years, with a risk of phones being lost, stolen or donated with EPHI on the device.[134] HIPAA security considerations are encryption of both the data at rest and data in transit, recipient authentication, and auditing controls (e.g., ability to record and examine system activity to determine if a security violation occurred).[135] Each practice must do risk analysis when considering texting, weighing patient care considerations against security concerns. Some opt for secure text messaging applications; others opt to use text for appointment reminders only. Policies and procedures should address this issue for the workforce.

Emailing. The Security Rule does not specifically forbid use of email for sending EPHI. Transmission security is an addressable requirement, so it is incumbent upon the practitioner to decide if unencrypted emails adequately protect EPHI. A solution must be selected, a decision made, the decision documented.[136] Some practitioners decide to not communicate any EPHI via email, while others set limits on what may be communicated via email (e.g., only appointment confirmations). Some give the patient the opportunity to agree or object to in their informed consent, educating about the potential for breach of their EPHI. Emails sent within the workforce on an internal server are considered secure (though there is still a risk of an internal message being sent to the wrong person). For both texting and emails, policies and procedures should detail the CE's specific rules on the issue. Access control, integrity, and transmission security should all be considered.

Summary

HIPAA does not specify use of any particular technology, as the U.S. Department of Health and Human Services wanted to make electronic data safeguards as flexible as possible; this makes sense given fast-evolving cyber threats. No doubt the dance between cyber threats and cyber defenses will continue. In this chapter, we examined prevention and cure of cyber threats, the risks and benefits of social media, and explored the use of texting and emailing for rapid communication with patients and other providers. All efforts to contain a breach must be integrated into one's larger security program.

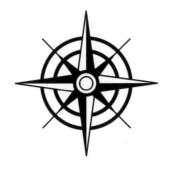

CHAPTER 15

Frequently Asked Questions

Q: Am I required to encrypt my emails?

A: It depends upon what you are emailing. First, encryption is an addressable specification. This means that you must implement what is "reasonable and appropriate" for your practice. However, remember that if data is lost, if it is encrypted, it falls under the "safe harbor" exemption and is not considered a breach. Data in transit is most at risk; if you are sending Electronic Protected Health Information (EPHI), yes, you should encrypt, though technically you are not required to since encryption is addressable specification. If you are sending records, you can easily encrypt through Winzip. Your other option is to put the document on a secure server that is encrypted. There are many options such as Google drive, Go Daddy, Drop Box, among others. Windows 7 and 10 have included full drive encryption within the software. Another option is to save your document as a PDF and subsequently encrypt it.

Q: I do not do electronic billing, but I do fax documents. Do I need to be HIPAA compliant?

A: No, faxing in and of itself does not make you a covered entity (CE).

However, you may be subject to other regulations around the privacy and security of PHI.

Q: What about text messages?

A: Under the regulations, clients have the right to request alternate methods of communication. If the client requests to communicate through text messages, you should explain the risks, and have them acknowledge the risks and sign permission for the alternate form of communication. If a patient texts you, it is reasonable to assume that they understand the risks, but additional explanation of potential risks is prudent.

If text messages are being sent between two providers, and they contain PHI, the texts should to be encrypted, though this is an addressable standard so the provider has discretion to establish what is "reasonable and appropriate." If a text is sent that is nebulous such as "your 4:00 canceled," you do not need to encrypt.

Q: How do I know I am getting reliable information about HIPAA?

A: You want to look at the quality of credentials of the consultant, company, or author. Many people claim expertise and either do not have credentials or have done a few hours of training. Certain credentials require a rigorous exam, much like a licensing exam. The following are excellent credentials:

ORGANIZATION	CERTIFICATION
American Health Information Management Association (AHIMA)	Certified in Healthcare Privacy and Security (CHPS)
Healthcare Information and Management Systems Society (HIMSS)	Certified Associate in Healthcare Information and Management Systems (CAHIMS) Certified Professional in Healthcare Information and Management Systems (CPHIMS)
Information Systems Audit and Control Association (ISACA)	Certified Information Systems Auditor (CISA) Certified Information Security Manager (CISM) Certified in Risk and Information Systems Control (CRISC) Cybersecurity Nexus (CSX Certificate) & (CSX-P Certification)
(ISC)² (Inspire, Secure, Certify)	Certified Information Systems Security Professional (CISSP) Certified Health Care Information Security and Privacy Practitioner (HCISPPsm)
International Association of Privacy Professionals (IAPP)	Certified Information Privacy Professional (CIPP)

Table 15.1. HIPAA related training credentials

Q: Why do I need HIPAA anyway?

A: This is a common question. We all must take common sense steps to keep patient information private. This includes privacy, but also security of EPHI. Anyone who has had their identity stolen can vouch for why this is important!

Q: How often do I need to do a security risk assessment (SRA)?

A: There is not a statutorily defined time period. Common best practice is to do it annually. If there is a material change to your operations or technology structure you want to re-assess. If you have a breach, you must also re-assess your security.

Q: What are my obligations for training?

A: While most people do an annual training on general HIPAA requirements, the regulations require that you train on specific policies and procedures relative to each workforce member's job. While many practitioners opt to purchase e-learning on HIPAA, training needs to be on *your own* practice's, policies and procedures, not just general knowledge of HIPAA. Every workforce member needs to be trained within a reasonable period of time when they join your organization; for sensitive information such a psychotherapy information, training should occur before access to PHI. You also need to train anytime that you have a breach.

Q: My electronic health records vendor says that they are HIPAA compliant. Doesn't that take care of my HIPAA requirements?

A: Organizations are HIPAA compliant, not specific technology. HIPAA requires you to do a security risk assessment as well as due diligence on your business associates (BAs) to be sure they are following HIPAA regulations. BAs are required to monitor compliance of their subcontractors.

Q: What should I do if I get a subpoena?

A: Make sure it is a valid subpoena, and be sure you document information released in your accounting of disclosures. You must attempt to ensure (1) that the patient has been given notice of the request (and a chance to respond), or you must secure a qualified protective order, which prohibits the parties from disclosing the protected health information (PHI) for any other purposes than litigation and (2) that the PHI be returned to the CE or destroyed at the end of the litigation. It is always prudent to have an attorney review the subpoena.

Q: I understand that HIPAA allows for disclosure of some psychotherapy information, but not psychotherapy notes. However, my state requires a patient's consent to release any mental health information. Did HIPAA erode patient privacy rights?

A: No. You are allowed to obtain patient consent to use or disclose their PHI, allowing you to stay consistent with your state law.

Q: How do I know what businesses I work with qualify as business associates (BAs), and which do not?

A: A BA is any person or organization who does work for you, who is not a workforce member and who has access to paper or electronic PHI. Any of your employees or volunteers are not BAs. Anyone who is on the treatment team (e.g., other therapists, referring physicians, supervisors) are not BAs. Additionally, janitors, cleaning staff, and repair persons are not considered BAs, and do not require a BA agreement.

Q: All I have is one computer, why do I have to worry about doing an security risk assessment?

A: If you are doing electronic billing, you are a CE, subject to the HIPAA privacy and security regulations, which includes performing the security risk analysis. HIPAA is considered the gold standard for security of PHI. By following HIPAA regulations, you provide yourself with an affirmative defense when a breach occurs.

Q: How do I know if I am HIPAA compliant?

A: A quick assessment of compliance consists of being able to (1) readily pull out your HIPAA policy and procedures manual; (2) produce your training logs (who was trained, when they were trained, a copy of the training materials, and who provided the training), (3) produce your security risk assessment, and (4) produce your consequent remediation plan; and, (5) evidence that you have done due diligence on your BAs. These five items are only the forerunners of what you will be required to provide the Office for Civil Rights as part of a breach investigation or random audit.

Q: Can we have a sign-in sheet in our waiting room?

A: Yes, seeing a name on the sign-in sheet is considered an "incidental disclosure" and not a breach of PHI. However, many CEs add additional security by having the patient sign on a peel off label, which they remove when the person has signed in. Alternatively, others simply redact (black out) the name of the patient after they have checked in.

Q: Does the size of my practice affect my HIPAA compliance?

A: All CEs must follow the privacy regulations. However, the Department of Health and Human Services allows CEs to consider their size, capabilities, and costs when determining what specific security measures to use to protect PHI.

Q: I am confused by the concept of "minimum necessary." Does everyone in my practice get only the minimum necessary information regarding patients?

A: Minimum necessary does not apply when disclosures are needed for treatment purposes, when releasing information to the patient or their representative, or when a patient authorizes release of PHI, or in other situations required by law. If staff are not involved in treatment of a patient, they should get the minimum necessary information required for them to do their job.

Q: Does HIPAA require me to submit my claims electronically?

A: No, you are not required to submit your claims electronically, though some government benefit programs (e.g., Medicare) require electronic submission of claims. Additionally, other third-party payers may require you to submit claims electronically.

Q: Is it acceptable to Skype with patients?

A: This has been a hotly debated topic. The answer is, yes Skype is acceptable IF you purchase Skype for business AND enter into a BAA with Microsoft. Additionally, the American Telemedicine Association offers guidelines for video-based online mental health services (www.americantelemed.org) that suggests other secure options. Encryption standards are available through the National Institute of Standards and Technology (NIST).

Q: In my practice, everyone uses their personal cell phones. Is this ok?

A: Because mobile devices are highly prone to loss or theft, they should be encrypted (again this is an addressable requirement so CEs must decide what is "reasonable and appropriate"). The practice should have policies and procedures addressing lockout features, appropriate use of texting, appropriate use of camera and video, the ability to examine the mobile device for compliance, and a requirement that the phone can be remotely wiped. Strong power-on passwords are suggested, as well as screen locks when the device is not in use. Additionally CEs need to be sure all EPHI is securely wiped at the end of the use of the phone, or when a workforce member leaves the employ of the CE.

Q: I am confused by all of the response times and storage times required by HIPAA. Can you clarify?

A: Table 15.2 reflects the most common response and storage times.

Patient requests their records	The CE must respond within 30 days (unless state law is stricter).
Patient requests to amend their records	The CE must respond within 60 days. One 30-day extension is permitted, but patient must be notified in writing with reason and expected response date.
Patient requests an Accounting of Disclosures	You must respond within 60 days. One 30-day extension is permitted, but patient must be notified in writing with reason and expected response date.
HIPAA Complaints	This complaint must be filed within 180 days of when the complainant knew or should have known that the act had occurred. The secretary may waive this 180-day time limit if good cause is shown. Complaints must be maintained for six years.

Denials of Access to Patient Records	Patients are not privy to psychotherapy notes, and information compiled for legal proceedings (unless state law allows). PHI that was obtained from someone other than the provider under the promise of confidentiality may be denied when access would reveal the source of the information or when access could lead to harm. Denials must be made within 30 days.
Retention of HIPAA Policies and Procedures	Policies and procedures should be kept six years from the date they were created or were last in effect, whichever is later.
Notice of Privacy Practices	A CE must provide a Notice of Privacy Practices (NPP) no later than the date of first service delivery, unless it is an emergency. If there is an emergency, the NPP may be provided as soon as reasonable after the emergency. If there are changes to an NPP, the latest version must be available for individuals to request to take with them, and it must be posted prominently at the facility.
Records Retention for Treatment Records	HIPAA defers to state law on this issue.
Policies and Procedures	Policies and procedures must be kept six years from the date of their creation, or the date when they were last in effect, whichever is later.

Breach Notification	Without unreasonable delay and no later than 60 days following the discovery of a breach (or within 60 days of the discovery of a breach of a BA)

Table 15.2. Response times and data storage requirements

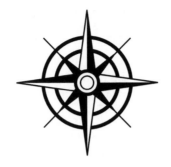

APPENDIX A

Model Notice of Privacy Practices for
Mental Health Professionals

Our Responsibilities

- We are required by law to maintain the privacy of your health information.

- We will let you know promptly if a breach of your health information occurs that may have compromised the privacy or security of your information.

- We must follow the duties and privacy practices described in this notice unless you tell us otherwise in writing. If you do so, you may change your mind at any time (you must provide notification of this change to us in writing).

- We are required to abide by the terms of this notice until we officially adopt a new notice. We will provide a copy of the new notice.

- We are required to give you a copy of this notice.

Your Rights as a Patient

- **You have the right to get a copy of your paper or electronic medical record** unless state law prohibits it. You may ask to see or receive an electronic or paper copy of your medical record and other information we may have about you. Upon request, we will provide you a copy or a summary of your health information typically within 30 days of your request. You will be charged a reasonable, cost-based fee.

- **To ask us to correct your medical record.** If you believe your medical record is incorrect or incomplete you may ask us to correct it. We have the right to decline your request, but we must do so in writing within 60 days.

- **You have the right to ask us to contact you in a specific way.** For example, you may want to be contacted at a specific phone number or to send your mail to an alternate address.

- **You have the right to ask us to limit what we share with others.** For example, you can ask us not to share certain health information that we use for treatment, payment, or business operations. We are not required to grant this request; we may decline your request if we believe it would affect your care.

- **You have the right to ask for a list of the times we have shared your health information, who we have shared it with, and why.** This accounting of disclosures of information can be for up to six years prior to the date you ask. The accounting will include all disclosures except for those we have made about your treatment, payment, or healthcare operations, and certain other disclosures, such as those you requested that we make. You are able to receive one such accounting per year; after that, we will charge a reasonable cost-based fee if you ask for another accounting

- **You have the right to request not to share information with your insurer if you pay for services out of pocket.** If you pay for services in full yourself, you can ask that we not share that information with your health insurer.

- **You have the right to ask for a paper copy of this notice at any time.** We will promptly provide it.

- **You have the right to choose a personal representative.** If you have given someone medical power of attorney or if you have a legal guardian, that person may exercise your rights and make choices about your health information. We will try to make sure this person has the proper authority prior to disclosing your health information.

- **You have the right to agree or object to our sharing of your health information under certain conditions.** For example, you can tell us if you would like us to share information with your family, friends, or others involved in your care. You may also choose to tell us if you would like your health information shared in the event of a disaster so, for example, family or friends could locate you. In the event of an emergency and you are unable to tell us your preferences for these matters, we will use our professional judgement and share information if we believe it is in your best interest.

- **You have the right to opt out of fundraising solicitations.** We may contact
you regarding fundraising efforts, but you may opt-out and tell us not to contact you again.

- **You have the right to complain if you believe your privacy rights have been violated.** We cannot retaliate should you file a complaint.

How We Use Your Health Information

What follows are exceptions to your confidentiality; the health information may be disclosed without your consent. Information that is disclosed in these situations will be kept to the minimum to meet the requirement or to the extent required by law.

We will use your health information in the following way:

- **For Your Treatment.** We may use your health information and share it with other professionals who are treating you. For example, a clinician treating you may need to speak with a psychiatrist or another clinician seeking input to increase the quality of your care.

- **For Payment.** We may use and disclose your health information in order to receive payment for services you obtain from us. For example, we may give limited information to your insurance company or other payer for billing and payment purposes.

- **For Our Healthcare Operations.** We may use and disclose your health information for administrative purposes. For example, we may use your healthcare information for quality assessment and improvement functions, evaluating your clinician, or accreditation or licensing activities.

Other Uses and Disclosures of your Health Information

We can also share health information about you for certain situations such as:

- Reporting suspected abuse, neglect, or domestic violence
- Preventing or reducing a serious threat to anyone's health or safety
- For workers' compensation claims (as the law allows)
- Reporting adverse reactions to medications
- Complying with the law
- For health research
- Preventing disease
- Helping with product recalls
- For law enforcement purposes or with a law enforcement official as indicated or allowed by law
- With health oversight agencies for activities authorized by law
- For special government functions such as military, national security, and presidential protective services
- Responding to lawsuits and legal actions

- In response to a court or administrative order, or in response to a subpoena
- To family members involved in your care unless you have objected
- With a personal health representative whom you have designated
- For research purposes if certain conditions are met
- Responding to organ and tissue donation requests
- Working with a coroner, medical examiner, or funeral director
- For certain specialized government functions (e.g. prisons, military)
- To Business Associates (Certain services are performed through contract with outside persons or organizations. Our Business Associates abide by written contracts that obligates them to safeguard your information in the same manner we do.)

Special Protections for Your Psychotherapy Notes

- Your psychotherapy notes are afforded additional protections under the law. Psychotherapy notes are "notes recorded (in any medium) by a mental health professional documenting or analyzing the contents of conversation during a private counseling session or a group, joint, or family counseling session." Psychotherapy notes are kept separate from your medical record. Psychotherapy notes do not include treatment information including medication prescription and monitoring, counseling session start and stop times, the modalities and frequencies of treatment furnished, results of clinical tests, and any summary of the following items: Diagnosis, functional status, your treatment plan, symptoms, prognosis, and progress. These may be included in your medical record and may be used to carry out treatment, payment, or our healthcare operations as discussed above.
- Your psychotherapy notes will not be released without your express written permission, except under the following circumstances: by the healthcare provider who created the notes for oversight purposes, when needed by the coroner or medical examiner, or when needed to avert a serious and imminent threat to health or safety of yourself or others. In the event of legal action against us, we may use your psychotherapy notes to defend ourselves in legal proceedings.

How We Will *Not* Use Your Protected Health Information

- We will not use your protected health information for marketing purposes without your written permission.
- We will not share psychotherapy notes in most cases without express written authorization from you.
- We will not sell your health information.

Minors in Treatment

- Minor's privacy is regulated by state law. <FILL IN YOUR STATE LAW>

If You Believe Your Privacy Rights Have Been Violated

If you believe your privacy rights have been violated, you have the following rights:

- You may complain to us if you feel we have violated your rights by contacting our Privacy Officer at <INSERT PHONE, EMAIL, MAILING ADRESS OF YOUR ORGANIZATION>.
- You may also file a complaint with the U.S. Department of Health and Human Services Office for Civil Rights by sending a letter to 200 Independence Avenue, S.W., Washington, DC 20201, or by calling 1-877-696-6775, or vesting www.hhs.gov/ocr/privacy/hipaa/complaints/. <You are not required to include this statement in your NPP; it is optional.>

You may revoke this authorization at any time in writing. For any further information needed, please contact our Privacy Officer at <INSERT CONTACT INFORMATION>.

Changes to the Terms of This Notice: We can change the terms of this notice, and the changes will apply to all information we have about you. The new notice will be available upon request, in our office, and on our web site.

Effective date, April 14, 2013

This notice was adapted from the model at hhs.gov.

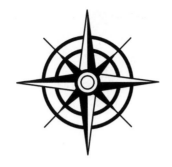

APPENDIX B

Sources of Help

- HHS HIPAA information: www.hhs.gov

- HHS phone: 866-627-7748

- To sign up for privacy or security listserves: www.hhs.gov/hipaa/for-professionals

- Compliance Assistance: www.hipaacomplianceusa.net

- Health Insurance Portability and Accountability Act Collaborative of Wisconsin (HIPAA COW): www.hipaacow.org

- American Health Information Management Association: www.ahima.org

- Gasch, A., & Gasch, B. (2010). Protecting your patient data. *In Successfully Choosing Your EMR: 15 Crucial Decisions.* Hoboken, NJ: Wiley-Blackwell.

- National Institute for Standards and Technology: www.csrc.nist.gov

- State Law: www.alllaw.com

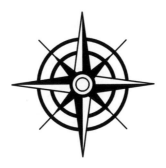

GLOSSARY

Access: the ability or means to read, write, modify, or communicate protected health information or otherwise use any system resource.

Access authorization: policies and procedures that determine which individuals in the workforce have access to electronic protected health information.

Access control: ensures that only users with rights or privileges to access and perform functions using information systems, applications, programs, or files.

Access controls and validation procedures: procedures to control and validate a person's accessibility to facilities based on their role or function, including visitor control, and control of access to software programs for testing and revision.

Access establishment and modifications: policies and procedures that establish, review, and modify a workforce member's right to access a workstation, transaction, program, or process.

Accountability: a record of movements of electronic media or hardware housing electronic protected health information.

Accounting of disclosures: a report that records when the medical center discloses a patient's private health information for purposes other than treatment, payment, or healthcare operations.

Addressable: a covered entity can evaluate how to implement a HIPAA-addressable implementation specification, implement an equivalent alternative measure that allows the entity to comply with the standard, or not implement the addressable specification or any alternative measures if equivalent measures are not reasonable and appropriate within its environment.

Administrative safeguards: administrative actions, policies, and procedures to manage the selection, development, implementation, and maintenance of security measures to protect electronic protected health information and to manage the conduct of the covered entity's workforce in relation to the protection of that information.

Administrative simplification: national standards for privacy protections for individually identifiable health information.

American Recovery and Reinvestment Act (ARRA) of 2009: an act enacted in part to promote the adoption and meaningful use of health information technology; American Recovery and Reinvestment Act brought the Health Information Technology for Economic and Clinical Health Act.

AOD: Accounting of Disclosures

Applications and data criticality analysis: an analysis that will prioritize the software applications (data applications that store, maintain, or transmit electronic protected health information) and data that are most important to patient needs and must be restored first in the event of a disaster or emergency operations.

ARRA: the American Recovery and Reinvestment Act of 2009

Audit: an independent examination or adjustment of accounts to ensure compliance with the HIPAA Privacy, Security, and Breach Notification Rules.

Audit controls: a process that monitors the hardware, software, and/or procedural mechanisms that record and examine activity in information systems that contain or use electronic protected health information.

Authentication: procedures to verify that a person or entity seeking access to electronic protected health information is the one claimed.

Authorization (HIPAA authorization): an individual's signed permission to allow a covered entity to use or disclose the individual's protected health information that is described in the authorization for the purpose(s) and to the recipient(s) stated in the authorization.

Automatic logoff: electronic procedures that terminate an electronic session after a predetermined time of inactivity.

BA: business associate.

Backup: the procedure in which documents are saved in case the original is lost or damaged.

Breach: an unauthorized use or disclosure under the HIPAA regulations that compromises the security of the protected health information.

Breach notification rule: the HIPAA Breach Notification Rule, requires HIPAA-covered entities and their business associates to provide notification following a breach of unsecured protected health information.

Business associate (BA): a person or organization that performs a function (such as billing, subcontracting, actuarial, or legal services) or activity on behalf of a covered entity, but is not part of the covered entity's workforce.

Business associate agreement (BAA) contract : an agreement between a HIPAA covered entity and a HIPAA business associate that ensures that health information is private and secure.

CE: covered entity.

Confidentiality: an ethical (and typically legal) obligation on the part of a mental health professional to not disclose private information.

Contrary: a term that indicates a covered entity would find it impossible to comply with both the state and federal requirements.

Contingency operations: categorization and prioritization of types of potential threats and vulnerabilities that might have an effect on facility access and develop policies and procedures that provide protection from threats and alleviate vulnerabilities.

Contingency plan: a plan for responding to a system emergency that includes performing backups, preparing critical facilities that can be used to facilitate continuity of operations in the event of an emergency, and recovering from a disaster.

Covered entity (CE): health plans, health care clearinghouses, and health care providers who electronically transmit any health information in connection with transactions for which the Department of Health and Human Services has adopted standards.

Consent: when an individual agrees to treatment by a health care provider.

CPT: Current Procedural Terminology.

Cure: remediating a breach to decrease damage caused to individuals.

Current Procedural Terminology (CPT): a widely accepted medical nomenclature system used to report medical procedures and services to health insurers.

Data authentication: the ability for an organization to provide corroboration that data in its possession has not been altered or destroyed in an unauthorized manner.

Data backup plan: a documented and routinely updated plan to create and maintain, for a specific period of time, retrievable exact copies of information.

Data integrity: refers to the accuracy and consistency of data or information that is stored.

Data use agreement: an agreement used to establish the permitted uses and disclosures of the limited data set by a recipient, consistent with the purposes of the research.

Decryption: a process that reverses the encryption algorithm process and makes the plaintext available for further processing.

De-identified data: information that does not identify the individual and for which there are logical reasons to believe an individual can be identified, which is not considered protected health information.

Designated record set (DRS): group of records maintained by or for a covered entity that is used, in whole or part, to make decisions about individuals, or that is a provider's medical and billing records about individuals or a health plan's enrollment, payment, claims adjudication, and case or medical management record systems. It is also used to clarify what protected health information can be accessed and amended.

Department of Health and Human Services: see Health and Human Services.

Device and media controls: policies and procedures that govern the receipt and removal of hardware and electronic media that contain electronic protected health information, into and out of a facility, and the movement of these items within a facility.

Disaster recovery: the policies, process, and procedures that are implemented after a natural or human-induced disaster designed to help in the recovery or continuation of vital technology within an organization.

Disaster recovery plan: part of an overall contingency plan. The plan for a process whereby an enterprise would restore any loss of data in the event of fire, vandalism, natural disaster, or system failure.

Disclosure: the release, transfer, provision of, access to, or divulging in any other manner protected health information outside of the covered health care component holding the information.

Disclosure statement: a document that is usually required by state statute that requires a mental health professional to reveal their licensure status and educational background, among other requirements.

Disposal: implement policies and procedure to address the final disposition of electronic protected health information and/or the hardware or electronic media on which it is stored.

DRS: designated record set.

EDI: electronic data interchange.

EHR: electronic health record.

EIN: employer identification number.

Electronic data interchange (EDI): computer-to-computer transmission of business information (e.g., insurance approval and reimbursement information) in a standard format.

Electronic health record (EHR): an electronic version of a patient's medical history that is kept by a provider. Also known as the electronic medical record.

Electronic protected health information (EPHI): electronic health data protected under the Security Rule.

Electronic transmission: transmission via the Internet (wide-open), Extranet (using Internet technology to link a business with information only accessible to collaborating parties), leased lines, dial-up lines, private networks, and those transmissions that are physically moved from one location to another using magnetic tape, disk, or compact disk media.

Employer identification number (EIN): a 9-digit IRS employer identification number that must be used by covered entities with standard transactions.

Emergency access procedure: procedures for obtaining necessary electronic protected health information during an emergency.

Emergency mode operation: when a covered entity is operating in emergency mode due to technical failure or power outage, emergency mode operation is a security process to protect electronic protected health information that must be maintained.

Encryption: a process that combines plain text with other values called keys, or ciphers, so the data becomes unintelligible.

Entity authentication: the verification that the user of protected health information is who it claims to be.

GLOSSARY

EPHI: Electronic protected health information.

Evaluation: periodic reports considering both technical and nontechnical appraisals of security procedures.

Facility security plan: policies and procedures that safeguard a facility and the equipment therein from unauthorized physical access, tampering, and theft.

Final Omnibus Rule: a set of regulations issued by the Department of Human and Health Services in 2013 to modify the Health Insurance Portability and Accountability Act to implement provisions of the Health Information Technology for Economic and Clinical Health Act to strengthen privacy and security of individual's health information and modify the breach notification rule.

Firewall: part of a computer system or network that is designed to block unauthorized users from accessing information.

Health and Human Services: the department of the government that oversees the creation and implementation of the HIPAA regulations.

Health care clearinghouse (HCC): an entity that processes health information received in a nonstandard format into a standard format (with standard data elements for a standard transaction) or into a nonstandard format (with nonstandard data content) for a receiving entity.

Health care operations: certain administrative, financial, legal, and quality improvement activities of a covered entity that are necessary to run its business and to support the core functions of treatment and payment.

Health Information Technology for Economic and Clinical Health Act (HITECH): enacted as part of the American Recovery and Reinvestment Act of 2009, with the purpose of promoting the adoption and meaningful use of health information technology. It also established penalties and fines for breaches of protected health information.

Health plan: any provider of medical or other health services, or supplies, who transmits any health information in electronic form in connection with a transaction for which the Department of Health and Human Services has adopted a standard.

Health plan identifier: a 9-digit unique identifier for reimbursement entities.

Health care provider: a provider of services, a provider of medical or other health services, and any other person who furnishes or bills and is paid for health care services or supplies in the normal course of business.

Health Insurance Portability and Accountability Act (HIPAA): regulations enacted in part to protect the privacy and security of private health information.

Hybrid entity: a covered entity whose business activities include both covered and noncovered functions.

ICD: The International Classification of Diseases, a medical classification code set that is a diagnostic tool for classifying diseases, often used for reimbursement purposes.

Implementation specification: a more detailed description of the method or approach covered entities can use to meet a particular security standard.

Incidental use and disclosure: a secondary use or disclosure that cannot reasonably be prevented, is limited in nature, and occurs as a result of another use or disclosure that is permitted by the HIPAA regulations. An example is when a patient inadvertently hears another patient's name during scheduling of an appointment.

Individual: means the person who is the subject of the protected health information.

Individually identifiable health information: any information, including demographic information, collected from an individual that is created or received by a health care provider, health plan, employer, or health care clearinghouse and relates to the past, present, or future physical or mental health or condition of an individual, the provision of health care to an individual, and identifies the individual or there is a reasonable basis to believe that the information can be used to identify the individual.

Information access management: formal, documented policies and procedures for granting different levels of access to health care information.

Information system: an interconnected set of information resources under the same direct management control that shares common functionality. A system normally includes hardware, software, information, data, applications, communications, and people.

Informed consent: a consent that describes the risks and benefits of treatment; it is not required by HIPAA regulations.

Integrity controls: implement security measures to ensure that electronically transmitted electronic protected health information is not improperly modified without detection until disposed of.

Internal audit: an in-house review of the records of system activity (such as logins, file accesses, and security incidents) maintained by an organization.

Intrusion detection: a type of security management system for computers and networks that observes security-related events, notifies security administrators of the events that should be analyzed further, and produces reports for evaluation.

LDS: limited data set.

LHR: legal health record.

Limited data set (LDS): protected health information from which certain specified direct identifiers of individuals and their relatives, household members, and employers have been removed.

Legal health record (LHR): a covered entity decides which health care documents constitutes their official record for evidentiary purposes which serves to support the decisions made of the patient's care or justification for third-party payment.

Log-in monitoring: policies and procedures for monitoring login attempts and detecting and reporting discrepancies.

Maintenance records: policies and procedures that document repairs and modifications to the physical components of a facility that are related to security.

Malicious software: software created to gain unauthorized control of another computer.

Mechanism to authenticate electronic protected health information: mechanisms to substantiate that electronic protected health information has not been altered or destroyed in an unauthorized manner.

Media controls: controls that govern the receipt and removal of hardware/software (e.g., CDs, USBs) into and out of a facility.

Media reuse: addresses the final disposition of electronic protected health information and/or the hardware or electronic media on which it is stored, as well as to implement procedures for removal of electronic protected health information from electronic media before the media are made available to be used again.

Medical identity theft: unlawful use of another person's identity for purposes such as an individual fraudulently receiving medical services, prescription drugs, and/or goods.

Memorandum of understanding (MOU): when a covered entity and a business associate are both government entities, they may draw up a formalized statement of mutual expectations between the two agencies.

Minimum necessary: the minimum information a covered entity should reveal when satisfying a particular purpose or carrying out a function (e.g., uses and disclosures).

Minimum necessary standard: The minimum necessary standard requires covered entities to evaluate their practices and enhance safeguards as needed to limit unnecessary or inappropriate access to and disclosure of protected health information. Protected health information should only be viewed to the extent that it is needed to satisfy a particular purpose or carry out a function.

Mitigation: reducing, to the extent practicable, any harmful effects that are known to the covered entity that result from use or disclosure of private health information in violation of its own privacy policies and procedures or the HIPAA regulations.

Modifications: changes to the HIPAA rules by the Department of Health and Human Services.

More stringent: When a state law provides greater privacy protections for individuals' identifiable health information, or greater rights to individuals with respect to that information than does the Privacy Rule. State laws are "more stringent" when they prohibit or restrict disclosures that are otherwise allowed under HIPAA.

MOU: memorandum of understanding.

National Institute of Standard and Technology (NIST): a federal agency that is responsible for developing standards and guidelines, including minimum requirements, used by federal agencies in providing adequate information security for the protection of agency operations and assets.

National plan and provider enumeration system: a branch of the Department of Health and Human Services that provides unique identification numbers for providers, employers, and health plans.

National provider identifier: a unique identification number for covered entities.

NIST: National Institute of Standard and Technology.

Notice of Privacy Practices (NPP): a notice that protects the rights of an individual by providing a clear, user-friendly explanation of with respect to their personal health information and the privacy practices of health plans and health care providers.

NPP: Notice of Privacy Practices.

Office for Civil Rights: the federal entity that carries out its enforcement responsibilities of HIPAA regulations.

OCR: Office for Civil Rights.

Organized Health Care Arrangement (OHCA): an arrangement that agrees a patient's private health information can be shared in order to manage and benefit between two or more covered entities who participate in joint activities.

Password management: procedures for creating, changing, and safeguarding passwords.

Payment: encompasses the various activities of health care providers to obtain payment or be reimbursed for their services and of a health plan to obtain premiums, to fulfill their coverage responsibilities and provide benefits under the plan, and to obtain or provide reimbursement for the provision of healthcare.

Periodic security reminders: electronic, paper, or oral reminders of security concerns to the workforce on an ongoing basis.

Person or entity authentication: procedures to verify that a person or entity seeking access to electronic protected health information is the one claimed.

Personal representative: the individual who has the ability to act for the individual and exercise the individual's rights.

Phishing: an cyber attempt to access personal information, typically involving an email or text solicitation which resembles a legitimate business or person; the goal of phishing is to steal personal information or introducing malware to procure your personal information.

Physical access controls: formal, documented policies and procedures for limiting physical access to an entity while ensuring that properly authorized access is allowed.

Physical safeguards: physical measures, policies, and procedures to protect a covered entity's electronic information systems and related buildings and equipment, from natural and environmental hazards, and unauthorized intrusion.

PHI: protected health information.

Policies and procedures standard: reasonable and appropriate policies that cover administrative, physical, and technical safeguards.

Privacy: the right to not have your personal information divulged to others without your permission.

Privacy official: the individual in an organization responsible for developing and implementing privacy policies and procedures and serves as (or designates) a contact person or contact office responsible for receiving complaints and providing individuals with information on the covered entity's privacy practices.

Privacy Rule: establishes national standards that require safeguards to protected health information, setting limits and conditions on uses and disclosures of patients PHI.

Protected health information (PHI): any information, whether oral or recorded, in any form or medium that (1) is created or received by a health care provider, health plan, public health authority, employer, life insurer, school or university, or health care clearinghouse and (2) relates to the past, present, or future physical or mental health or condition of an individual, the provision of health care to an individual, or the past, present, or future payment for the provision of health care to an individual.

Protection from malicious software: covered entities must assure that its systems and data are safe and secure from unauthorized access that might lead to the alteration, damage, or destruction of automated resources and data, unintended release of data, and denial of service.

Psychotherapy notes: particularly sensitive information that includes the personal notes of the therapist that typically are not required or useful for treatment, payment, or health care operations purposes, but only for use by the mental health professional who created the notes.

Required: means that a covered entity must implement the security standard or specification.

Risk analysis: an assessment of the potential risks and vulnerabilities to the confidentiality, integrity, and availability of electronic protected health information held by the covered entity, also known as a security risk assessment.

Risk management: implementation of security measures sufficient to reduce risks and vulnerabilities to a reasonable and appropriate level.

Risk mitigation: involves taking early action to prevent or reduce the likelihood of risk to security of protected health information.

Role-based access: each workforce member is assigned to one or more predefined roles, each of which has been assigned the various privileges needed to perform that role.

Safeguards: ensure the integrity and confidentiality of protected health information and protect against any reasonably anticipated threats or hazards to the security or integrity of the information and unauthorized use or disclosure of the information.

Sanction policy: covered entities must apply appropriate sanctions against workforce members who fail to comply with the security policies and procedures of the covered entity.

Scalability: refers HIPAA allowing covered entities to analyze their own needs and implement solutions appropriate for their specific environments. This includes size, complexity, capabilities, technical and hardware infrastructure, and costs of security measures.

Security: a health care provider's responsibility to prevent to unauthorized disclosure, destruction, or loss of electronic protected health information.

Security awareness and training: training program for all members of its workforce (including management), which includes periodic security reminders, user education and protection from malicious software, log-in monitoring, and password management.

Security incident: a violation or imminent threat of violation of computer security policies, acceptable-use policies, or standard computer security practices.

Security incident response and reporting: requires a covered entity to identify and respond to suspected or known security incidents, mitigate, to the extent practicable, harmful effects of security incidents that are known to the covered entity, and document security incidents and their outcomes.

Security management process: a process designed to implement policies and procedures to prevent, detect, contain, and correct security violations.

Security official: the person designated to oversee development and implementation of policies and procedures that safeguard electronic protected health information.

Security reminders: periodic security updates disseminated to the workforce.

Security risk assessment (SRA): an assessment of the potential risks and vulnerabilities to the confidentiality, integrity, and availability of electronic protected health information held by the covered entity.

Security Rule: requires administrative, physical, and technical safeguards to protect electronic protected health information.

Spear phishing: phishing with the target being a specific individual or business.

SRA: security risk assessment.

Standards: regulations set by HIPAA to ensure appropriate administrative, physical, and technical safeguards to ensure the confidentiality, integrity, and security of electronic protected health information.

Standard unique employer ID: a nine digit employer identification numbers assigned by the Internal Revenue Service, which must be used in standard transactions between payers and providers.

Subcontractor: an entity that creates, receives, maintains, or transmits protected health information on behalf of a business associate.

Technical safeguards: defined as the technology and the policy and procedures for its use that protect electronic protected health information and control access to it.

Technology neutral: a security standard is "technologically neutral," meaning no specific technologies are required by the regulations, in order to facilitate the use of the latest and most promising technologies.

Termination procedures: a covered entity must implement procedures for terminating access to electronic protected health information when the employment of a workforce member ends.

Testing and revision procedures: procedures for periodic testing and revision of contingency plans.

Threat: the potential for a person or thing to exercise (accidentally trigger or intentionally exploit) a specific vulnerability.

TPO: treatment, payment, and health care operations.

Transaction: the exchange of information between two parties to carry out financial and administrative activities related to health care.

Transmission security: security measures that guard against unauthorized access to electronic protected health information when data is being transmitted electronically.

Treatment: the provision, coordination, or management of health care and related services among healthcare providers or by a health care provider with a third party, consultation between health care providers regarding a patient, or the referral of a patient from one health care provider to another.

Unique user identification: a unique name and/or number for identifying and tracking user identity for workforce who have access to electronic protected health information, so that system access and activity can be identified and tracked by user.

Unsecured protected health information: protected health information that is not secured through the use of a technology to render protected health information unusable, unreadable, or indecipherable to unauthorized individuals.

Use: with respect to individually identifiable health information, the sharing, employment, application, use, examination, or analysis of such information within an entity that maintains such information.

User: a person or entity who has access to medical records that contain private health information.

User authentication: an assigned unique name and/or number for identifying and tracking user identity.

User-based access: restrict access to electronic protected health information based on the workforce member's identity.

Vulnerability: potential flaw or weakness in a covered entity or business associate security procedures.

"Wall of Shame": a breach portal maintained by the Department of Health and Human Services that reports any significant breaches of protected health information by a covered entity or business associate, including the amount of individuals affected, and the type of location of the breach.

Whaling: a phishing attack aimed at a senior official in an organization or business.

Willful neglect: conscious, intentional failure or reckless indifference to the obligation to comply with the HIPAA regulations.

Workforce: employees, volunteers, trainees, and other persons whose conduct, in the performance of work for a covered entity, is under the direct control of such entity, whether or not they are paid by the covered entity.

Workforce clearance procedure: procedures to determine that the access of a workforce member to electronic protected health information is appropriate.

Workforce security: policies and procedures that ensure that all members of the workforce have appropriate access to electronic protected health information and prevent those workforce members who do not have access under from obtaining access to electronic protected health information.

Workstation: an electronic computing device, for example, a laptop or desktop computer, or any other device that performs similar functions, and electronic media store in its immediate environment.

Workstation use: policies and procedures to protect electronic protected health information by safeguarding the physical surroundings of electronic devices housing electronic protected health information.

Workstation security: physical safeguards that restrict access to electronic protected health information to authorized users.

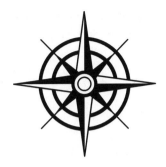

ENDNOTES

1. For consistency, I use the word *patient* throughout the book, understanding that you may use the word *client* depending upon whether or not you are ensconced in the medical model.

2. For access to state statutes, go to www.alllaw.com (see " state law resources")

3. See http://criminal.findlaw.com/criminal-rights/is-there-a-difference-between-confidentiality-and-privacy.html for more information on confidentiality and privacy.

4. Federal Trade Commission. (2007). 2006 Identity theft survey report: Prepared for the Commission by Synovate. Retrieved from https://www.ftc.gov/reports/federal-trade-commission-2006-identity-theft-survey-report-prepared-commission-synovate

5. Ibid.

6. HHS. (n.d.). The Privacy Rule. Retrieved from http://www.hhs.gov/ocr/privacy/hipaa/administrative/privacyrule/

7. HHS. (n.d.). The Security Rule. Retrieved from hhs.gov/hipaa/forprofessionals/security/

8. HIPAA, Public Law 104-191, 5 C.F.R. §160.103.

9. Popken, B., & Grant, K. (2015, February 15). Anthem hack: Millions of non-anthem customers could be victims. Retrieved from http://www.nbcnews.com/tech/security/anthem-hack-millions-non-anthem-customers-could-be-victims-n312051

10. Pepitone, J. (2015). Premera blue cross hacked: 11 million customers could be affected Premera blue cross hacked: 11 million customers could be affected . Retrieved from http://www.nbcnews.com/tech/security/premera-blue-cross-hacked-11-million-customers-affected-n325231

11. Privacynet. (2015). Aspire Indiana notifies over 45,000 employees and clients after burglars nab office laptops. Retrieved from http://www.phiprivacy.net/?s=aspire+&searchsubmit=

12. Davis, H. (2013). Laptop with patient info stolen from employee's home. Retrieved from http://www.yumasun.com/laptop-with-patients-info-stolen-from-home/article_71ff7535-ff5d-5aa3-afa4-8a2e70f89a2c.html

13. Bosworth, M. (2006). Mental health clinic loses laptop bearing patient data, *Consumer Affairs*. Retrieved from http://www.consumeraffairs.com/laptop-data-theft

14. Health Privacy Project. (2003). Medical privacy stories. Retrieved from http://patientprivacyrights.org/wp-content/uploads/2013/08/True_Stories1.pdf

15. PHIPrivacy.net. (2013). Comprehensive Psychological Services in South Carolina had a laptop stolen which included psychological records and custody evaluations. Retrieved from http://www.phiprivacy.net/psychological-assessments-provider-notifies-patients-after-laptop-with-phi-stolen-in-office-burglary/

16. HHS. (n.d.). HIPAA settlement underscores the vulnerability of unpatched and unsupported software. Retrieved from http://www.hhs.gov/ocr/privacy/hipaa/enforcement/examples/acmhs/index.html

17. HHS. (n.d.). HHS settles with health plan in photocopier breach case. Retrieved from http:// www.hhs.gov/ocr/privacy/hipaa/enforcement/examples/affinity-agreement.html

18. HHS. (n.d.). Alaska DHSS settles HIPAA security case for $1,700,000. Retrieved from http://www.hhs.gov/ocr/privacy/hipaa/enforcement/examples/alaska-agreement. html

19. Dimick, C. (2010). Californian sentenced to prison for HIPAA violation. *Journal of the American Health Information Management Association*. Retrieved from http://journal.ahima.org/2010/04/29/californian-sentenced-to-priHson-for-hipaa-violation/

20. Dimick, C. (2008). Arkansas HIPAA violator sentenced. *Journal of the American Health Information Management Association*. Retrieved from http://journal.ahima.org/2008/12/08/arkansas-hipaa-violator-sentenced/

21. Information Security Media Group, Inc. (2015). Prison term in HIPAA violation case. *InfoRiskToday*. Retrieved from http://www.inforisktoday.com/prison-term-in-hipaa-violation-case-a-7938/op-1

22. American National Standards Institute (2012). The financial impact of breached protected health information. Retrieved from webstore.ansi.org/phi

23. Ponemon Institute. (2013). Cost of data breach study. Retrieved from https://www4.symantec.com/mktginfo/whitepaper/053013_GL_NA_WP_Ponemon-2013-Cost-of-a-Data-Breach-Report_daiNA_cta72382.pdf

24. HHS. (n.d.). U.S. Department of Health and Human Services Office for Civil Rights Breach Portal: Notice to the Secretary of HHS Breach of unsecured protected health information. Retrieved from https://ocrportal.hhs.gov/ocr/breach/breach_report.jsf

25. Hecker, L.L., & Edwards, A.A. (2014). The impact of HIPAA and HITECH: New standards for confidentiality, security, and documentation for marriage and family therapists, *American Journal of Family Therapy, 42* (2), 95-113, doi: 10.1080/01926187.2013.792711

ENDNOTES

26. Acosta v. Byrum, 180 N.C. App. 562, 638 S.E.2d 246 (North Carolina, 2006).

27. Loria, G. (2015). HIPAA Breaches: Minimizing Risks and Patient Fears Industry View. Retrieved from http://www.softwareadvice.com/medical/industryview/hipaa-breaches-report-2015/

28. HHS. (2013). HHS announces first HIPAA breach settlement involving less than 500 patients: Hospice of North Idaho settles HIPAA security case for $50,000. Retrieved from http://www.hhs.gov/news/press/2013pres/01/20130102a.html

29. Sanches, L. (2012). 2012 HIPAA privacy and security audits. *National Institute of Standards and Technology*. Retrieved from http://csrc.nist.gov/news_events/hiipaa_june2012/day2/day2-2_lsanches_ocr-audit.pdf

30. *Jaffee v. Redmond et al.*, 1996 WL 315841 (U.S. June 13 1996).31HIPAA, Public Law 104-191, 45 C.F.R. §160.501

31. HIPAA, Public Law 104-191, 45 CFR §160.103

32. Minnesota Department of Health, Office of Health Information Technology. (2014). HIPAA, Minnesota's Health Records Act, and Psychotherapy Notes. Retrieved from http://www.health.state.mn.us/e-health/privacy/ps102114psychotherapy.pdf

33. HIPAA Collaborative of Wisconsin (COW). (2015). Use and disclosure of psychotherapy notes policy. Wisconsin HIPAA COW Privacy Networking Group. Retrieved from http://hipaacow.org/wp-content/uploads/.../HCR-Psychotherapy-Notes-FINAL-5-11-15.doc

34. OH Matters. (2015). RG, UO Senate, Prof. Freyd all unimpressed by Coltrane's leadership on sexual assaults. Retrieved from http://uomatters.com/2015/03/rg-uo-senate-prof-freyd-all-unimpressed-by-coltranes-leadership-on-sex-assaults.html

35. Foden-Vencil, K. (2015). College rape case shows a key limit to medical privacy. *National Public Radio*. Retrieved from http://www.npr.org/sections/health-shots/2015/03/09/391876192/college-rape-case-shows-a-key-limit-to-medical-privacy-law

36. *Jaffee v. Redmond et al.*, 1996 WL 315841 (U.S. June 13 1996).

37. HIPAA, Public Law 104-191, 45 C.F.R. Parts 160 and 164 (Subparts A and E).

38. HHS (n.d.). All case examples: Mental Health Center Corrects Process for Providing Notice of Privacy Practices. Retrieved from http://www.hhs.gov/ocr/privacy/hipaa/enforcement/examples/allcases.html

39. HHS. (2003). Frequently asked questions: Must a covered entity revise the whole notice every time one state law materially changes? Retrieved from http://www.hhs.gov/hipaa/for-professionals/faq/464/must-a-covered-entity-with-a-notice-revise-the-notice-every-time-it-changes/index.html

40. HHS. (2014). Health information privacy: Model Notice of Privacy Practices. Retrieved from http://www.hhs.gov/ocr/privacy/hipaa/modelnotices.html

41. Ibid.

42. Ibid.

43. Ibid.

44. Ibid.

45. Dougherty, M. (2001). Accounting and tracking disclosures of protected health information (AHIMA Practice Brief). *Journal of AHIMA, 72* (10), 72E-H. Retrieved from http://library.ahima.org/xpedio/groups/public/documents/ahima/bok1_009468. hcsp?dDocName=bok1_009468

46. 45 CFR Part 160, Part 164 (Subparts A and C).

47. HHS. (2007). HIPAA Security Series, Security Standards: Administrative Safeguards, *Security Series, 2* (paper 3). Retrieved from http://www.hhs.gov/ocr/privacy/hipaa/administrative/securityrule/adminsafeguards.pdf

48. HHS. (2007). HIPAA Security Series, Security Standards: Physical Safeguards, *Security Series, 2* (paper 2). Retrieved from http://www.hhs.gov/ocr/privacy/hipaa/administrative/securityrule/physsafeguards.pdf

49. HHS. (2007). HIPAA Security Series, Security Standards: Technical Safeguards, http://library.ahima.org/doc?oid=300266#.V1ICRvkrLX42 (paper 4). Retrieved from http://www.hhs.gov/ocr/privacy/hipaa/administrative/securityrule/techsafeguards.pdf.48 HHS. (2014). Security risk assessment. *Security Series 2* (paper 6). Retrieved from http:// www.healthit.gov/providers-professionals/security-risk-assessment

50. HHS (n.d.). Final guidance on risk analysis. Retrieved from http://www.hhs.gov/hipaa/for-professionals/security/guidance/final-guidance-risk-analysis/index.html

51. National Institute for Standards and Technology. (2011). NIST Special Publication 800- 39 Managing information security risk. Retrieved from http://csrc.nist.gov/publications/ nistpubs/800-39/SP800-39-final.pdf

52. HealthIT.gov (2014). Security Risk Assessment. Retrieved from https://www.healthit.gov/providers-professionals/security-risk-assessment

53. National Institute for Standards and Technology. (2011). NIST Special Publication 800- 39 Managing information security risk. Retrieved from http://csrc.nist.gov/publications/ nistpubs/800-39/SP800-39-final.pdf

54. Walsh, T. (2013, November). Security risk analysis and management: An overview (2013 update). AHIMA Practice Brief. Retrieved from http://library.ahima.org/doc?oid=300266#.V1ICRvkrLX4

55. Wheeler, E. (2011). *Security risk management: Building an information security risk management program from the group up.* Waltham, MA: Elsevier.

56. National Institute for Standards and Technology. (2011). NIST Special Publication 800- 39 Managing information security risk. Retrieved from http://csrc.nist.gov/publications/ nistpubs/800-39/SP800-39-final.pdf

57. HHS. (2007). Basics of Risk Analysis and Risk Management. *Security Series, 2* (paper 6). Retrieved from http://www.hhs.gov/ocr/privacy/hipaa/administrative/securityrule/riskassessment.pdf

58. Wheeler, E. (2011). *Security risk management: Building an information security risk management program from the ground up.* Waltham, MA: Elsevier.

59. Ibid.

60. Ibid.

61. Ibid.

62. Ibid.

63 Walsh, T. (2013, November). Security risk analysis and management: An overview (2013 update). *AHIMA Practice Brief.* Retrieved from http://library.ahima.org/doc?oid=300266#.V1ICRvkrLX4

64 Adapted from Wheeler, E. (2011). *Security risk management: Building an information security risk management program from the group up.* Waltham, MA: Elsevier.

65. National Institute of Standards and Technology. (2012). NIST Special Publication 800-30 (rev. 1), Guide for conducting risk assessments. Retrieved from http://csrc.nist.gov/publications/nistpubs/800-30-rev1/sp800_30_r1.pdf

66. Wheeler, E. (2011). *Security risk management: Building an information security risk management program from the group up.* Waltham, MA: Elsevier.

67. Snedaker, S. (2013). Risk mitigation strategy development. In S. Snedaker's *Business Continuity and Disaster Recovery Planning for IT Professionals,* (pp. 337–367). New York, NY: Elsevier, Inc.

68. Wheeler, E. (2011). *Security risk management: Building an information security risk management program from the ground up.* Waltham, MA: Elsevier.

69. Snedaker, S. (2013). Risk mitigation strategy development. In S. Snedaker's *Business Continuity and Disaster Recovery Planning for IT Professionals,* (pp. 337–367). New York, NY: Elsevier, Inc.

70. HHS (2015, September 2). $750,000 HIPAA settlement emphasizes the importance of risk analysis and device and media control policies. Retrieved from http://www.hhs.gov/about/news/2015/09/02/750,000-dollar-hipaa-settlement-emphasizes-the-importance-of-risk-analysis-and-device-and-media-control-policies.html

71. HHS Office of the National Coordinator for Health Information Technology and Office for Civil Rights. (2012). Security Risk Assessment. Retrieved from http://www.healthit.gov/providers-professionals/security-risk-assessment.

72. National Institute of Standards and Technology. (2012). NIST Special Publication 800-30 (rev. 1), Guide for Conducting Risk Assessments. Retrieved from http://csrc.nist.gov/publications/nistpubs/800-30-rev1/sp800_30_r1.pdf.

73. Wheeler, E. (2011). *Security risk management: Building an information security risk management program from the ground up.* Waltham, MA: Elsevier.

74. Lambert, B. & Schweber, M. (2007, Oct 10). Hospital workers punished for peeking at Clooney file. *New York Times.* Retrieved from http://www.nytimes.com/2007/10/10/nyregion/10clooney.html?_r=0

75. Gorman, A., & Sewell, A. (2013, July 12). Six people fired from Cedars-Sinai over patient privacy breaches. *Los Angeles Times*. Retrieved from http://articles.latimes. com/2013/jul/12/local/la-me-hospital-security-breach-20130713

76. HHS. (2005). Security Standards: Administrative Safeguards. *HIPAA Security Series, 2*. Retrieved6fromhttps://www.infinisource.com/media/6881/HIPAA%20Security%20 Series%202--Administrative%20Safeguards%20(CMS).pdf

77. Ibid.

78. HHS Office of the National Coordinator for Health Information Technology and Office for Civil Rights. (2012). Security Risk Assessment. Retrieved from http://www. healthit.gov/providers-professionals/security-risk-assessment

79. National Institute of Standards and Technology. (2012). NIST Special Publication 800-30 (rev. 1), Guide for Conducting Risk Assessments. Retrieved from http://csrc.nist. gov/publications/nistpubs/800-30-rev1/sp800_30_r1.pdf

80. HHS (2013).HHS settles with health plan in photocopier breach case.Retrieved from https://wayback.archive-it.org/3926/20150618191048/http://www.hhs.gov/news/ press/2013pres/08/20130814a.html

81. Health Privacy Project. (2003). Health privacy stories. Retrieved from https://www. cdt.org/files/healthprivacy/20080311stories.pdf

82. HHS Office of the National Coordinator for Health Information Technology and Office for Civil Rights. (2012). Security Risk Assessment. Retrieved from http://www. healthit.gov/providers-professionals/security-risk-assessment

83. National Institute of Standards and Technology. (2012). NIST Special Publication 800-30 (rev. 1). Guide for Conducting Risk Assessments. Retrieved from http://csrc.nist. gov/publications/nistpubs/800-30-rev1/sp800_30_r1.pdf

84. Daily News (2009, March 31). 15 workers fired for accessing octuplet mom Nadya Suleman's file. Retrieved from http://www.nydailynews.com/entertainment/gossip/15-workers-fired-accessing-octuplet-mom-nadya-suleman-file-article-1.362031

85. National Institute of Standards and Technology. (2012). NIST Special Publication 800-30 (rev. 1). Guide for Conducting Risk Assessments. Retrieved from http://csrc.nist. gov/publications/nistpubs/800-30-rev1/sp800_30_r1.pdf

86. Masters, G. (2008). Nation's first encryption law. Retrieved from http://www. scmagazine.com/nations-first-encryption-law/article/120402/

87. AHIMA. (2001, March). Security audits of electronic health information (Updated). *Journal of AHIMA, 82* (3), 46–50.

88. AHIMA. "The 10 Security Domains (Updated 2013)." *Journal of AHIMA 84* (10) (October 2013): expanded web version. Retrieved from http:// library.ahima.org/xpedio/ groups/public/documents/ahima/bok1_050430. hcsp?dDocName=bok1_050430

89. HHS. (2007). Security standards: Organizational, policies and procedures and documentation requirements. *HIPAA Security Series, 2*, paper 5.

90. Under Organizational Requirements, there are also requirements for group health plans to comply with appropriate safeguards, protect the security of epHI, and document as such 45 CFR §164.314(b)(1).

91. Washington Post (2006, May 22). U.S. says personal data on millions of veteran's stolen. Retrieved from http://www.washingtonpost.com/wp-dyn/content/article/2006/06/29/AR2006062900352.html

92. HIPAA, Public Law 104-191, 45 CFR Parts 160, 162, and 164.

93. Ponemon Institute. (2014). Fourth annual benchmark study on patient privacy and data security. Retrieved from http://www.ponemon.org/blog/fifth-annual-benchmark-study-on-patient-privacy-and-data-security

94. Ibid.

95. Ibid.

96. Brinda, D. (2016, Februrary 22). 2015 healthcare data breaches: paper tops data breach location! Retrieved from http://www.tripointhealthcaresolutions.com/2015-healthcare-data-breaches-paper-tops-data-breach-location/

97. Walgreen Co v. Abigail E. Hinchey, App. Ct. Ind., Nov. 14, 2014 (Indiana, 2014).

98. Web, G. (August, 2002). Avoiding a HIPAA Nightmare: An unbelievable example of what can go very wrong. Retrieved from http://www.gilweber.com/resources/journal-articles-and-essays/avoiding-a-hipaa-nightmare/

99. HIPAA Journal. (n.d.). The HIPAA wall of shame: Major data breaches of 2013. Retrieved from http://www.hipaajournal.com/hipaa-wall-shame-major-data-breaches-2013/

100. Ibid.

101. PHIprivacy.net. (2013). Emmorton associates notify patients after locked file cabinet with counseling records broken into. Retrieved from http://www.phiprivacy.net/?s=emmorton&searchsubmit=

102. PHIPrivacynet. (2012). Choices, Inc. hacked: clients' SSN and health info accessed. http:// www.phiprivacy.net/choices-inc-hacked-clients-ssn-and-health-info-accessed/

103. McCann, E. (2014, October 14). Email hack leads to data breach. Healthcare IT News. Retrieved from http://www.healthcareitnews.com/news/hipaa-breach-letters-go-out-after-email-hack

104. McCann, E. (2014, May 19). Keylogger hack at root of HIPAA breach. *Healthcare IT News*. Retrieved from http://www.healthcareitnews.com/news/keylogger-hack-root-hipaa-breach

105. Compliagent Solutions. (2015). Recent HIPAA Violations: 5 Largest HIPAA Breach Fines since 2009. Retrieved from http://www.compliagent.com/blog/2015/1/27/recent-hipaa-violations-5-largest-hipaa-breach-fines-since-2009

106. Rose, D. & Batista, S. (2010). Attorney: Doctor to notify 900 patients about discarded records. Retrieved from http://www.wbtv.com/story/12715146/attorney-doctor-to-notify-900-patients-about-discarded-records

107. McGee, M.K. (2013, August 9). Secure Disposal of Data: Lessons Learned. Retrieved from http://www.govinfosecurity.com/blogs/secure-disposal-data-lessons-learned-p-1532

108. NBC News. (2015). Anthem hack: Millions of non-anthem customers could be victims. Retrieved from http://www.nbcnews.com/tech/security/anthem-hack-millions-non-anthem-customers-could-be-victims-n312051

109. National Institute for Standards and Technology. (2014). NIST Cryptographic Standards and Guidelines Development Process. Retrieved from http://www.nist.gov/public_affairs/releases/upload/VCAT-Report-on-NIST-Cryptographic-Standards-and-Guidelines-Process.pdf

110. AHIMA. (2013). Performing a breach risk assessment. *Journal of AHIMA*, 84(9), 66–70.

111. International Conference on Information Security and Artificial Intelligence. (2013). 10 crazy cases of identity theft. Retrieved from http://www.isai2010.org/10-crazy-cases-of-identity-theft/

112. Ponemon Institute. (2015). Fifth annual benchmark study on patient privacy and data security. Retrieved from https://www2.idexpertscorp.com/fifth-annual-ponemon-study-on-privacy-security-incidents-of-healthcare-data.

113. Jenkins, M.K. (2013). The "dirty dozen" healthcare IT issues. *Journal of the American of the American Association for Orthopaedic Surgeons*. Retrieved from http://www.aaos.org/AAOSNow/2013/Nov/managing/managing9/?ssopc=1

114. HHS Cybersecurity Program (2015). Information systems security awareness training. Retrieved from http://docplayer.net/1262280-The-department-of-health-and-human-services-information-systems-security-awareness-training-fiscal-year-2015.html.

115. Ibid.

116. Malenkovich, S. (2013, January 16). How attackers actually steal data. *Kaspersky Lab Daily*. Retrieved from https://blog.kaspersky.com/how-attackers-actually-steal-data/933/

117. Siciliano, R. (2013, July 23). What is a keylogger? Consumer, family safety, identity protection, mobile security consumer log: McAfee. Retrieved at https://blogs.mcafee.com/consumer/what-is-a-keylogger/

118. Grebennikov, N. (2007, March 29). Keyloggers: How they work and how to detect them. Secure List. Retrieved from https://securelist.com/analysis/publications/36138/keyloggers-how-they-work-and-how-to-detect-them-part-1/

119. Sage, A. (2014, August 19). New HIPAA breach leader on HHS Wall of Shame. Retrieved from https://www.linkedin.com/pulse/20140819200723-7839522-new-hipaa-breach-leader-on-hhs-wall-of-shame

120. HHS Cybersecurity Program (2015). Information systems security awareness training. Retrieved from http://docplayer.net/1262280-The-department-of-health-and-human-services-information-systems-security-awareness-training-fiscal-year-2015.html

121. HHS (2015). Summaries of the Office of the Chief Information Officer (OCIO) policies, standards, and charters. Retrieved from http://www.hhs.gov/ocio/policy/ociosummaries.html

122. HHS Cybersecurity Program (2015). Information systems security awareness training. Retrieved from http://docplayer.net/1262280-The-department-of-health-and-human-services-information-systems-security-awareness-training-fiscal-year-2015.html

123. NIST (2007). Guide to intrusion detection and prevention system (IDPS), Special Publication 800-94. Retrieved from http://csrc.nist.gov/publications/nistpubs/800-94/SP800-94.pdf

124. HHS (n.d.). Health information privacy: Guidance to render unsecured protected health information unusable, unreadable, or indecipherable to unauthorized individuals. Retrieved from http://www.hhs.gov/ocr/privacy/hipaa/administrative/breachnotificationrule/brguidance.html

125. Burdon, M., Reid, J., and Low, R. (2010). Encryption safe harbors and data breach notification laws. *Computer Law and Security Review*, 26, 520–534.

126. NIST (2007). Guide to Storage Encryption Technologies for End User Devices, publication 800-111. Retrieved from http://csrc.nist.gov/publications/nistpubs/800-111/ SP800-111.pdf

127. HHS (n.d.). Health Information Privacy: Is the use of encryption mandatory in the Security Rule? Retrieved from http://www.hhs.gov/ocr/privacy/hipaa/faq/securityrule/2001.html

128. Hyden, M. (2013). HIPAA and encryption technology: Don't let the fear of hackers blind you to likelier threats. *MGMA Connexion, 9*, 45–46.

129. Ponemon Institute. (2013). Cost of data breach: Global analysis. Retrieved from http://www.ponemon.org/blog/2013-cost-of-data-breach-global-analysis

130. Gasch, A., & Gasch, B. (2010). Protecting your patient data. *Successfully choosing your EMR: 15 Crucial Decisions*. Hoboken, NJ: Wiley-Blackwell.

131. HHS Cybersecurity Program. (2015). Information systems security awareness training. Retrieved from http://docplayer.net/1262280-The-department-of-health-and-human-services-information-systems-security-awareness-training-fiscal-year-2015.html

132. Ponemon Institute. (2013). Cost of data breach: Global analysis. Retrieved from http://www.ponemon.org/blog/2013-cost-of-data-breach-global-analysis

133. Insurion. (n.d.). Technology for professionals: Protecting data to minimize malpractice and other liability claims. Retrieved from https://alliedhealth.insureon.com/Portals/15/ images/hipaa-ebook/ebook_technology_mental_health_professionals.pdf

134. Collier, N. (2015). Keep text messaging secure. *For the Record*, 27(3), 25.

135. Ibid.

136. HHS. (n.d.). Health information privacy: Does the Security Rule allow for sending electronic PHI (e-PHI) in an email or over the Internet? If so, what protections must be applied? Retrieved from http://www.hhs.gov/ocr/privacy/hipaa/faq/securityrule/2006.html

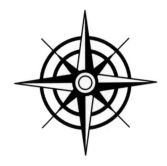

INDEX

Note: *f* represents a figure and *t* represents a table.

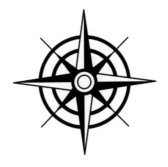

ABOUT THE AUTHOR

Lorna L. Hecker, Ph.D., LMFT, CHPS

Lorna is the Executive Vice President and Director of Education and Training at Carosh Compliance Solutions, a HIPAA compliance consultancy. Additionally, Lorna runs the company's professional practice in behavioral health. Lorna holds CHPS certification (certified in healthcare privacy and security) is through the American Health Information Management Association. Lorna is a frequent speaker on HIPAA topics unique to behavioral health practices.

In addition to HIPAA training and education endeavors at Carosh, Lorna is a professor of behavioral sciences at Purdue University Northwest, where she is on the faculty of the marriage and family therapy master's program. She is the director for the Purdue University Northwest Couple and Family Therapy Center. Lorna teaches graduate courses in professional and ethical issues, couples therapy, trauma, theories of family therapy, and play in family therapy, while maintaining a professional practice. Lorna has authored or edited nine books on various mental health topics, including ethics and professional issues, and has published articles and made national and international presentations in the field of mental health.

Made in the USA
Middletown, DE
08 September 2020